Protocols in Primary Care Geriatrics
Second Edition

Springer

New York
Berlin
Heidelberg
Barcelona
Budapest
Hong Kong
London
Milan
Paris
Santa Clara
Singapore
Tokyo

John P. Sloan

Protocols in Primary Care Geriatrics

Second Edition

With a Foreword by Mark Williams

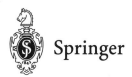 Springer

John P. Sloan, M.D.
Division of Community Geriatrics
Vancouver General Hospital
855 West 12th Avenue
Vancouver, BC V4Z IM9
Canada

Library of Congress Cataloging-in-Publication Data
Sloan, John P., M.D.
    Protocols in primary care geriatrics / John P. Sloan. — 2nd ed.
       p.   cm.
    Includes bibliographical references and index.
    ISBN 0-387-94690-X (soft)
    1. Geriatrics.   2. Medical protocols.   I. Title.
    [DNLM: 1. Geriatrics—case studies.   2. Primary Health Care.   WT
100 S6338p   1996]
    RC952.S56   1996
    618.97—dc20
    DNLM/DLC
    for Library of Congress   96-11918

Printed on acid-free paper.

Production coordinated by Chernow Editorial Services, Inc. and managed by
Terry Kornak; manufacturing supervised by Jeffrey Taub.
Typeset by Best-set Typesetter Ltd., Hong Kong.
Printed and bound by R.R. Donnelley, Harrisonburg, VA.
Printed in the United States of America.

9 8 7 6 5 4 3 2 1

ISBN 0-387-94690-X Springer-Verlag New York Berlin Heidelberg SPIN 10524878

Foreword

The striking increase in average life expectancy during the twentieth century rates as one of the major events of our time. We are in the midst of a social revolution—one rooted not in a new ideology, but in our changing population patterns. For the first time in human history, infants in fortunate nations like ours can expect to live well into their seventies and beyond.

This demographic revolution increases pressure on resources, as it also creates further social change and new opportunities for older persons. Such rapid changes have left most people "living in the past," with their generally negative attitudes about aging and elderly people. The same outmoded beliefs are embedded in many of our health care programs.

In our youth-oriented culture, most of us still view old people as physically decrepit or in rapid, inevitable decline. Mentally, they are viewed as forgetful or childish, with little ability to learn and adapt. Socially and economically, they are often considered a burden. With such stereotypes, where is the expectation and encouragement for their continuing capacity to enrich their own lives, and to enrich society?

These deep-seated cultural stereotypes do not describe accurately the "new wave" of elderly persons or their potential contributions to society. Today's aging individuals are mostly far from decrepit: fewer than 25 percent experience any disability and fewer than 5 percent are in nursing homes. Intellectually, given new opportunities to learn and grow, they thrive. Given suitable occupation, they work with zest and competence well beyond the traditional age of retirement. Many have an emotional maturity and the kind of wisdom that comes only with age. In short, chronological

v

age has virtually lost its meaning as a useful index of individual capacity.

To be sure, many old people have special needs for health care and other supports. But these cannot be provided knowledgeably without abandoning the old stereotypes, without a broader public understanding of today's elderly population and its potential relationship to the rest of society. Such understanding will bring recognition of the many ways our later years can be more a culmination of life than a prelude to death.

Clearly these cultural, social, and economic challenges cannot be solely addressed by the medical profession. Nevertheless, physicians are drawn into it with significant responsibilities to do what we can to address the acute and chronic needs of elderly people. It is within this context that I welcome John Sloan's second edition of *Protocols in Primary Care Geriatrics*.

This is a book about good doctoring to older people and their families. John Sloan is one of those thoughtful practitioners, with a gift of creative expression and a willingness to share his approach. His basic message is deceptively simple: that effective geriatric care is the skillful application of scientific principles. This application requires understanding key concepts and remembering useful features of the differential diagnosis. The numerous and witty mnemonics serve not only as memory aids but also as reflections of John Sloan's mental acuity. How to address, support, and reassure the human being who is the patient or the concerned family member while bringing modern technology to bear on the situation is John Sloan's message. He appropriately considers the history and physical examination as the cornerstone of his approach.

The first edition of this book was considered the "secret weapon" of many academic geriatricians. The outlines gave ready access to the content, and the cases were instructive exercises for junior learners. This second edition is a welcome update, with revisions that reflect changes in emphasis and new sections on abuse, difficult behavior, and teamwork.

This is a book that can be read by anyone concerned with helping elderly people. But it is aimed at busy practitioners who have to manage competing responsibilities. Clearly John Sloan has enjoyed his task—his sense of humor and clinical insight are inescapable. I hope the reader will be stimulated on this literary journey to cure occasionally, to relieve often, and to comfort always.

MARK WILLIAMS

How to Use This Book

This second edition is similar in form to the first. Each of the topics considered critical to adequate geriatric care by primary care physicians is developed as a prose chapter. Clinical exercises in follow-on question and answer format follow each chapter. Finally, an outline of each of the topics is presented. Readers familiar with the first edition will find the topic areas somewhat changed to reflect changes in emphasis that have occurred since the first edition was published. Drugs and specific therapies, as well as approaches to diagnosis, have been updated.

People learn in various ways. *Protocols in Primary Care Geriatrics* is directed at primary care physicians and others with an interest in developing their knowledge and skills in caring for frail elderly people. Its format is designed to accommodate various learning styles.

The first section contains discussions of various important topics in geriatrics, arranged in chapters. Those who learn best by reading, or who wish to read for interest, may find this section helpful. At the end of each chapter is a teaching exercise that seeks to test the knowledge and skills that have been covered in the chapter.

These exercises are usually case studies, followed by questions. Comments on the various possible answers are found in the section Responses to Clinical Exercises. These comments may be found following the instructions at the end of each answer. The learning exercises may help anyone who finds they learn best by doing. Reading them will also provide examples of and elaborations on the ideas presented in the chapters.

The second part of the book, entitled Notes on Geriatrics, is in fact an outline of Part One. It is intended for quick reference, for augmenting the reading of Part One, and for the benefit of readers who learn best by memorizing, particularly using mnemonics. Part Two is, however, written to be read, and readers with limited time may find it a succinct source of information. It is intentionally informal and colloquial in style.

Acknowledgments

As with the first edition, many people besides the author have contributed to making this book possible. Lynn Beattie, Mary Blake, Bill Dalziel, Azmina Dharamsi, Larry Dian, Jacquie Fraser, Judy Kelly, Bett Lauridson, Janet Martini, Grady Meneilly, Sheila Nolan, Chris Rauscher, Les Sheldon, and Sue Turgeon made suggestions and reviewed chapters. The book could not have been written without their help.

Medical Care of the Dying (a publication of the Victoria Hospice Society) and *Clinical Ethics* (Jonsen, Siegler, and Winslade) were particularly helpful as references.

These sources of inspiration and support should claim and receive credit for anything of value in the second edition. Its errors and shortcomings belong entirely to the author.

Contents

Foreword by Mark Williams   v
How to Use This Book   ix
Acknowledgments   xi

Introduction   1

Part I   Geriatrics Topics and Questions   3

A.   Basis for Practice
    1. Aging and Frailty   5
    2. Comprehensive Geriatric Assessment   11
    3. Prescribing in the Elderly   23

B.   Clinical Problems
    4. Mobility Failure   33
    5. Incontinence   39
    6. Cognitive Impairment   46
    7. Depression   54
    8. Abuse, Alcohol, and Automobiles   61
    9. Constipation, Fecal Incontinence,
       and Pressure Sores   70
    10. Difficult Behavior   78

C.   Special Topics
    11. The Team and Case Management   89
    12. Home Care and Caregiver Support   94
    13. Nursing Home Care   100
    14. Palliative Care   107
    15. Ethical Issues   113

Responses to Clinical Exercises   119

Part II   Notes on Geriatrics   147

Bibliography   197
Index   203

Introduction

Ten years have passed since a series of lectures, given to family practice residents at St. Vincent's Hospital in Vancouver, developed into a set of written notes; five years have passed since those notes were published in expanded form as the first edition of *Protocols in Primary Care Geriatrics*. Yet it seems that far more time has passed, so great and sweeping are the recent changes in health care and in primary care geriatrics.

Health care reform, with its pressing and legitimate emphasis on cost control, has brought the consideration of value for money into our priorities, in some cases for the first time. Care in the community has grown to stand beside institutional care as a legitimate venue for managing frailty. Advances in clinical practice have changed our approach to incontinence, depression, Parkinson's disease, heart failure, and many other clinical problems.

The more the venues and specific strategies of geriatrics change, the more valuable becomes a return to basic principles of clinical geriatrics and of health care. The history and physical examination persists as a critical and underused element of clinical evaluation, alongside high-tech diagnostic equipment and sophisticated clinical evaluation instruments. Extra time taken in the complex care of older people still results in a better and more helpful understanding of their problems.

Above all, the sympathy of one human being for another and the responsibility we feel to help older people as their lives become increasingly difficult continue to make our clinical work rewarding and exciting, no matter how repetitive and difficult it may sometimes seem. That great and growing task of the routine health care of older people is, as ever, the legitimate work of primary care professionals.

Scientific advances, teaching, and organization of academic and clinical programs will always fall to highly trained specialists, but excellent primary care is irreplaceable at the center of health maintenance for the huge majority of older people needing care.

This second edition, like the first, is written primarily for physicians. It may also be useful for other health professionals, caregivers, and administrators with an interest in the clinical side of geriatric care. It is aimed, in any case, to assist with primary care and to encourage intelligent accumulation of experience and instinct among its individual practitioners. May we continue constructively to criticize and evaluate the generalizations delivered to us by our academic colleagues, the more usefully and accurately to apply them in the particular cases of our patients.

Multidisciplinary as primary geriatric care must always be, there occasionally arises a worry over how to name the people we care for. Some doctors find importance in the word *patient*, while others prefer *client*. We find there isn't much in a name in this situation but that one may wish to switch from one word to another to fit in comfortably with prevailing usage or to provide a particular emphasis (calling an incompetent person an "adult," for example). This is the convention, or lack of it, that we have followed.

These are times of change and, some would say, trouble in the world of health care. Whatever situation has developed by the turn of this century, we believe that the professionals remaining as the clinical leaders and role models will still be those who find an ever-renewed source of stimulation among the very elderly and frail. They are the most needy and most awe-inspiring of patients. May we make the most of our opportunity to travel a short way at their side.

Part I   Geriatrics Topics and Questions

A. Basis for Practice

CHAPTER 1

Aging and Frailty

Youth is a ware that will not keep; for some reason, creatures age and die. The study of this process, its description and causes, and the difference between aging and disease are the province of gerontology, the academic sister of geriatrics. Here we look at gerontology briefly and then at frailty, the real-world consequence of getting old and infirm.

Demographics of Aging

This subject is dominated by the results of our recently acquired widespread longevity. Traditionally, a human population is represented by a pyramid shape, with youngest individuals (at the bottom) most numerous and very old ones (at the top) few and far between. This pyramid looks increasingly like a rectangle as modern industrial societies evolve. There is, in fact, a huge proportional increase in the most elderly group: those over the age of 85.

The result of this change, about to increase in the coming several decades with aging of the postwar population bulge, is that we are a society of older, and old, people. But who are the members of this new majority?

Characteristics of the Elderly

The proportion of women increases with age. Only 12% of centenarians are male. Because older people outlive spouses, families, and friends, they tend to be increasingly alone. Social isolation, although not a necessary consequence of aging, is prevalent.

The trend toward better education in the general population is now being observed in the elderly. Quitting school to work, a frequent necessity in the 1930s, occurred less toward mid-century. This has not yet translated, statistically, into affluence. The majority of elderly people receive low or below-average incomes, since sustained productive employment becomes rarer with age.

Most disturbing but quite consistent on average is the increase in disability with age. At age 65, only 5% of the North American population is disabled enough to be in a nursing home, but by age 85, the number is 22%. Some of this disability may be preventable or remediable, but the end of life is more often than not characterized by loss of capability.

Why Do We Age?

This ancient question may be close to being answered. Traditionally, two types of theories have been advanced. Genetic theories have focused on limitation of cell doubling, the running out of a biological clock, and the fulfillment of evolutionary function. Stochastic (probability) theories see aging as an accumulation of damage due to genetic error, mutation, toxins, and autoimmunity.

If natural selection provides a true explanation for biology, it would be difficult to imagine the persistence of a characteristic that repaired molecular damage due to the aforementioned stochastic factors beyond an age where external forces (such as predators and bad weather) would eliminate the majority of the population. Our wild ancestors, subject to falling rocks and murderous beasts, probably rarely survived beyond the age of 50. Cellular mechanisms that repaired molecular damage in people older than this would simply not have been selected for and, therefore, aren't part of our genetic repertoire.

The Changes of Normal Aging

Some authorities estimate that function deteriorates owing to normal aging, disease, and disuse, in roughly equal proportions. This would mean that one-third is preventable by some sort of conditioning.

Generally, as people age, they grow more unlike one another. This makes the following general statements about aging less meaningful for individuals, since each trend hides a wide range. Certain individuals may seem almost unaffected by aging changes, while others experience them very profoundly.

Sleep tends to be interrupted rather than continuous. Sexuality diminishes in both sexes, but there is some evidence that cultural influences create a self-fulfilling prophecy here. All major organ systems decline measurably in function but only on average. Renal function, for example, may be nearly normal or virtually dialysis-level, all without identifiable disease states.

Psychosocial Aging

Personalities appear not to change beyond age 30. Elderly people become more "set in their ways" in a sense and more like their younger selves, except that they're old. Successful psychosocial aging may involve keeping one's coping strategies current and effective by continued socialization and gaining more satisfaction from peaceful pursuits consistent with diminished biological and psychological capacity.

And then every so often we are astounded by a 90-year-old who has never accepted that aging implies decline (and has had the biological good luck not to have been proven wrong), whose life is a symphony of childlike innocence, adolescent emotion, and midlife productive stamina, all delivered with the huge conviction of experience. So there is something to look forward to, after all.

Successful Aging

If one-third of aging is due to disuse, and some proportion of disease is due to an unhealthy lifestyle, then much of aging would theoretically be preventable. Universal estrogen replacement might virtually eliminate fractures in elderly women, for example. The failure of the promise of diet to eliminate heart disease, however, suggests that healthy living may provide its benefits in part through a conviction that one is doing the right thing. It will take several decades to evaluate the effect of our current preoccupation with exercise and diet. Although some studies of exercise in the elderly are promising, a full-scale life-style revision of a very old person could be more disruptive and dangerous than beneficial.

Frailty

Among older people, many age successfully and then decline and die over a very short time. Many more, however, experience loss of function over a longer time and become the focus of most clinical geriatrics. The term *frail* is falling out of favor, perhaps owing to overuse. Some definition of the focus of clinical geriatrics is important, however, to identify who will receive our comprehensive care, be the focus of our programs, be evaluated in our research, and be included in payment schemes that encourage good geriatric care.

With advancing illness (defined as number of diagnoses, morbidity, expense of health care, amount of medication, etc.), disability increases slowly and then begins to worsen exponentially. One might see a frail person as someone with much morbidity who is therefore subject to a sudden large increase in disability with a relatively trivial advance in morbidity. The flu, a change in medication, or a fall with soft-tissue injuries can put an old person permanently in extended care; similar insults leave younger people unscathed. Figure 1.1 illustrates this idea.

Traditionally, the frail are the functionally dependent. Someone who requires assistance with activities of daily living is, at a first approximation, someone who can benefit from traditional geriatric care. The capacity to benefit from comprehensive geriatric health care might further define frailty and exclude extremely disabled people with end-stage dementia, who require assistance with feeding or who are comatose.

A model of frailty as a balance-type scale has also been proposed, in which resources, which assist with maintain-

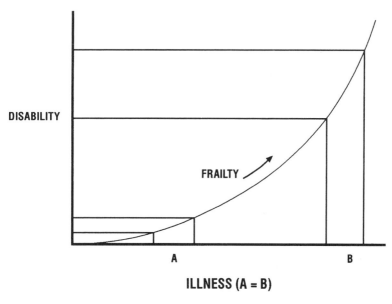

FIGURE 1.1. Frailty: The slippery slope (diagram courtesy David Brook, of Victoria, BC).

ing health, quality of life, and functional capacity, are piled on one side of the scale and liabilities, which lead to deterioration, rest on the other. When the scale is nearly in balance, interventions to decrease liabilities and strengthen resources can maintain stability. We would therefore focus our attention on patients whose assets and liabilities approximately balance.

A frail person requires attention. Support for activities of daily living is important, but surveillance to continually identify remediable problems as they arise is critical. Well-informed health professionals gradually change or augment their focus as frailty advances. Functional capacity and quality of life become more important than exact illness diagnosis and cure-oriented treatment as ends in themselves, important as they are. Evaluation of disease states and prescription of traditional curative interventions no longer necessarily contribute to the best outcome. Comprehensive geriatric assessment (see Chapter 2) is one method of applying the resources of health care to frailty.

Clinical Exercise

Try your hand at this question to test your knowledge of Chapter 1.

As far as we know, organisms, including humans, age because:

- There is a limited number of cell doublings, and once exhausted, that's it (turn to 1.1, page 119).
- Mutations, damage from free radicals and radiation, and autoimmune disease gradually accumulate (turn to 1.2, page 119).
- Human biology evolved at a time when lifespan was limited by external factors, so repairing of cell damage beyond age 50 doesn't make evolutionary sense (turn to 1.3, page 119).

Chapter 2

Comprehensive Geriatric Assessment

Every patient benefits most from the kind of evaluation and care suited to his or her problems. In psychiatry, it may be a mental status exam, formulation, and psychotherapy. In obstetrics, the obstetric history, fetal evaluation, and management of pregnancy, labor, and delivery are usual and most effective.

The frail elderly, whom we learned to identify in the first chapter, are best cared for by a system of information-gathering, evaluation, and ongoing care called *comprehensive geriatric assessment* (CGA). In this chapter, we look at the elements of this indispensable tool for the primary care geriatrics doctor. Using it, frail elderly people become manageable (if challenging); without it, their care can quickly get out of hand.

The process of CGA is about the same wherever it is applied. It can be used in the office, the nursing home, the patient's home, an acute care hospital, or a geriatric evaluation and management unit. Some venues are better suited than others, but even the fee-for-service family practice office can be tailored to permit thorough evaluation and care with a little creativity.

The frail elderly need two simultaneous points of view: a gestalt eyeball estimate of overall status and direction and a picky, exhaustive, detail-oriented approach embodying lists. They are, after all, complicated patients and have numerous problems that tend not ever to go away completely. Your care, aimed at maintaining independence and community support, is a continuing adjustment and readjustment exercise, in which the concept of a "stable" patient doesn't apply.

To do CGA properly you need plenty of help. Other professionals, family, and the patient become routinely involved in the enterprise. Comprehensive care can be understood and practiced in four basic steps.

Four Basic Steps

Figure 2.1 indicates the four "steps" on the circle of comprehensive geriatric assessment. First (at the top) baseline information is obtained. Next, a very thorough professional history and physical examination complete the data gathering process. The patient's problems and your ideas about dealing with them are next formulated, and then plans and a system for checking on intervention are put into place. This gathering of information, modifying the problem list, adjusting interventions, and taking a look back at the baseline function is the day-to-day business of primary care geriatrics. Ideally, the process is coordinated, and someone functions as the case manager by maintaining records, arranging and directing conferences, and deploying professionals and services.

Baseline

Three important pieces of information must be obtained to begin properly evaluating an older person: what is the level of function, degree of independence, or degree of disability?

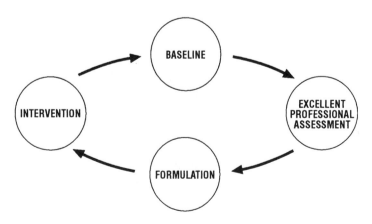

FIGURE 2.1. Four basic steps of comprehensive geriatric assessment.

Is the patient cognitively impaired, and if so, how badly? And what supports are in place and needed to achieve community independence?

Activities of Daily Living/Instrumental Activities of Daily Living (ADL/IADL)

Independence or function is measured in terms of activities of daily living (ADL) and instrumental activities of daily living (IADL). The capacity to perform these simple tasks is the precious resource that community geriatrics seeks to maximize and protect for the patient. Understanding the patient's abilities in these areas is as basic to their care as respiratory function in a chest patient or visual acuity for an ophthalmologist. As frailty advances, independence at ADLs fall off one by one.

The basic personal ADLs may be recalled using the mnemonic DEATH: dressing, eating, ambulating, toileting, and hygiene. Ambulating means mobility, which impacts on and affects other ADLs, and the IADLs. Hygiene would include bathing, brushing the teeth, and fixing the hair.

The IADLs are the tasks required for independent living, recalled by the mnemonic SHAFT: shopping, housework, accounting (banking), food preparation (cooking), and transport. Sometimes also included are laundry, medication taking, and use of the telephone.

Whether someone can perform each or any of these tasks may be difficult to evaluate precisely. Can I dress independently if it takes 70 minutes, if I need direction, or if I put my pants on backwards? The report of the patient or caregiver may be different from your impression when you objectively evaluate ADL performance.

It is hard to escape the fact, however, that an ADL or IADL that consistently cannot be performed must be supported (ie, done by someone else).

Cognition

Thinking capacity, or higher mental function, is often impaired in frail older people. Brain or cortical function is measured clinically as memory, orientation, calculation,

FOLSTEIN
MINI MENTAL STATUS EXAM

Date: _____   Examiner: _____

Score   ORIENTATION

(   )   What is the (year) (season) (month) (date) (day)   (5 pts)

(   )   Where are we? (country) (province) (city)   (5 pts)
                    (hospital) (floor)

                REGISTRATION

(   )   Name 3 objects: One second to say each. Then   (3 pts)
                    ask the patient to repeat all
                    three after you have said them.
                    One point for each correct.
                    Then repeat them until he
                    learns them. Count trials and
                    record _____

                ATTENTION AND CALCULATIONS

(   )   Serial 7s. One point for each correct answer. Stop
                at 5 answers. *Or* spell "world" backwards.
                (No. correct = letters before first mistake)   (5 pts)

                RECALL

(   )   Ask for the objects above. One point for each cor-   (3 pts)
                rect.

        (21)

                LANGUAGE TESTS
(   )   Name: pencil, watch   (2 pts)
(   )   Repeat: no ifs, ands, or buts   (1 pt)
(   )   Follow a three-stage command:
                "Take the paper in your right hand, fold it in half,   (3 pts)
                and put it on the floor."
(   )   Read and obey the following:
(   )   Close your eyes.   (1 pt)
                Write a sentence spontaneously below.   (1 pt)
(   )   Copy design below.   (1 pt)
        (9)

_____ Total (30 pts)

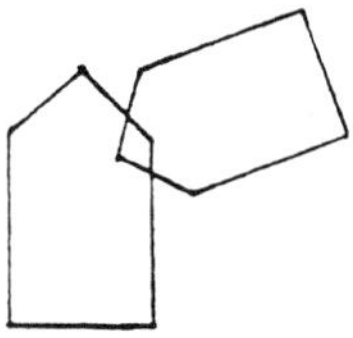

(   )

FIGURE 2.2. The Folstein Mini-Mental Status Examination.

insight, abstraction, and judgment; it is distinct from mood and thought disorders.

Unlike function (ADL/IADL), cognition is relatively easily and precisely measured, although there are still some problems with it. The most universally used instrument is the Folstein Mini-Mental Status Examination (Figure 2.2). The Short Portable Mental Status Questionnaire of Pfeiffer and more elaborate neuropsychological testing can also be used. "The Folstein" is a questionnaire giving a score out of 30 for higher mental function or cognition. Low intelligence, lack of education, anxiety, foreign language, and other cultural factors may alter the Folstein score. Still, there is definitely a difference between someone who scores 28 and someone who scores 21, and between someone who scores 19 and someone who scores 11.

Cognitively impaired people may have dementia, delirium, or both. Evaluation of attention and knowledge of the time course and fluctuations of the cognitive impairment will lead you to identify and promptly work up delirium, if it is present. The more demented the patient, the more difficult this becomes.

Social Supports

Your patient may tell you even less about the ADL/IADL supports in place than about the capability at doing the activities themselves. A collateral history from caregivers, neighbors, and others can be confirmed by your visit to assure that assistance with failed ADLs is in place.

Each activity a patient can't do must be done for him or her. Banking can be done by a trusted relative. Transportation may be available by community transit or through friends. A neighbor may shop. Dressing must be done twice daily and so is a more pressing need, as well as a less public one. People unable to transfer from bed to chair and to toilet independently or unable to eat a meal, need frequent care throughout every day.

Whoever gives this care is the caregiver, an extremely important individual to the patient. As frailty changes with illness and other health problems, caregivers may be stressed and overloaded. The primary care geriatrics case manager has the responsibility of supporting the supporters, and success at this means keeping flexible and preparing for changes. Someone housebound who needs daily assistance from spouse for dressing and meal preparation will end up, perhaps inappropriately, in an acute care hospital if pneumonia develops, unless the case manager is ready with temporary supports to assist with a sudden extra load.

ADL/IADL, cognition, and social supports form the community geriatrics baseline and are also the endpoints for care and treatment.

Excellent Professional Assessment

We call the community geriatrics history and physical examination excellent because second rate won't do. Frail elderly people have multiple problems, many systems are involved, data outside of traditional medicine, surgery, and psychiatry is required, and an improvement in health often results from a number of seemingly insignificant changes. A 20-minute "complete physical" that a well patient and routine family physician may consider adequate in the office doesn't even come close. The following mnemonics help to remind us of the history and physical points that must be added to the complete general medical evaluation we recall from our training. *Complete* is the operative word.

History ABCs

ADL/IADL. This reminds us, because the mnemonic is meant to stand alone, to evaluate function, which is also one of our baseline measurements.

Brain failure means cognitive impairment. Again, this baseline measurement must be made, but the history will include the time course, suggestions of delirium, and an evaluation of causes consistent with the history.

Collateral history. The patient seldom tells us the whole story. Family, caregivers, and other professionals must be approached for their versions. Sometimes collateral history is ongoing, and information about response to medication or other interventions comes from a spouse or caregiver.

Drugs and alcohol. Evaluation of medication must include compliance data. Unless compliance is ensured, medications and medication changes are even more dangerous than usual. Alcohol is often hidden and may present as withdrawal in a facility or acute care. See Chapters 3 and 8.

Emotional, behavioral, and psychological problems. This reminds us to evaluate carefully for past psychiatric history and to look for depression (common and often overlooked in older people), agitation and other behavior problems in demented people.

Falls and mobility failure. Problems with mobility may present as being chair- or bed-fast, or as falling or unsteadiness on one's feet. Specific questioning about the time course, safety, and about possible remediable causes (see Chapter 4) is essential.

Guardianship, caregiver, and placement. Impacting on ADL/IADL capability are the overriding issues of who looks after a frail person and where they live. Is the caregiver collapsing or abusive? Is the level of disability way beyond the type of domicile? Who is looking after the money?

Hazards. Make sure that appliances and smoking do not endanger the patient or neighbors. Safety behind the wheel is critical (see Chapter 8), and suggestions of neglect or active mistreatment can help you identify inappropriate caregiving and replace it.

Incontinence. Urinary and fecal problems may make caregiving difficult, destroy dignity, and be amenable to treatment.

Physical Evaluation ABCs

Expand the physical examination to include objective information gathering that gives a comprehensive picture:

Ambulation. This central ADL must be assessed with an objective measurement of balance and a good look at gait.

The "Get Up and Go" test (see Chapter 4) is a good standard evaluation. Look at safety and try to gather hints about the mobility failure diagnosis.

Blood pressure (BP) changes. Orthostatic hypotension is common and disabling. Check BP in two positions minimum. Significant orthostatic hypotension is symptomatic orthostatic hypotension.

Central nervous system (CNS) and musculoskeletal system (MSK). We are reminded that the two systems least frequently examined in the office are critical to older people's function. Power, deep tendon reflexes, coordination, and tone should be screened, looking for focal weakness, cerebellar disease, and Parkinsonism. The major joint range of movement, presence of pain, visible deformity and inflammation can be evaluated quickly in screening for disabling musculoskeletal problems.

Cognition (there are 3 Cs in this mnemonic). Chapter 6 outlines the quantitative evaluation of cognition. Normally, this means the Folstein Mini-Mental Status Examination, but more sophisticated testing may be necessary.

Competence. Legal considerations may require you to evaluate the patient's ability to manage his or her finances or to care for him or herself. If someone is to be appointed as a guardian, objective evaluation of the patient's performance at the task to be replaced is necessary. It is also important for you to take instructions on degrees of intervention (questions such as cardiac arrest resuscitation and hospital transfer) from a person capable of understanding the issues and instructing you meaningfully.

Drug-taking and alcohol evidence. Count pills to verify compliance. Alcohol odor, laboratory abnormalities, and bottles at home may supply information the history didn't disclose.

Environment. Loose carpets, no tub grab-rail, poor lighting, and broken stairways begin a long list dear to the occupational therapist's heart. Common sense is helpful here.

Function. Test ADL/IADL performance, and compare it to the report you got in the history. Some tests are indirect. Weight loss that reverses when meals are provided suggests shopping or cooking impairment, even if it is denied.

Formulation

Now that all the information is in, the elderly person's health profile can be listed comprehensively, now and for future reference. Leave no stone unturned. The comprehensive problem list may run to 8 or 20 items. It should state the problems in the most precise terms available. "Painful left leg, no diagnosis," "old left parietal infarct," "caregiver stress," are typical examples. Include past problems, functional problems, suspected problems, and unevaluated complaints.

The next step is to look at each of the problems in the comprehensive problem list and determine which ones might usefully be illuminated by further evaluation and possibly be amenable to intervention. Experience suggests that certain conditions are high-yield in this regard. Parkinson's disease, depression, multiple interacting medications, caregiver burnout, and mechanical foot problems are examples of disabling problems that are sometimes remediable. Dementia, left hemiplegia, well-investigated incontinence, and hypotension in severe well-treated angina and congestive heart failure would be problems likely not amenable to treatment. The remediable problem list contains the basis for the things you will attempt to do to assist your elderly patient with achieving stable, independent function.

Intervention

Normally one doesn't treat the frail elderly or evaluate the outcome of treatment alone. The facility nurse, the continuing care case manager, the family, the home care physiotherapist, adult day center supervisors, and others may be involved. Try to begin intervention by gathering a "team" together and making a common plan. Do your interventions, return to evaluate the outcome, and get together again to talk it over. This process continues as long as the patient remains in your care. Remember that its success is measured by its impact on the baseline: ADL/IADL, cognition, and appropriate supports in place.

The frail elderly are unpredictable and always changing. With a detailed and accurate baseline, supports in place, plans for crisis intervention, and a group of professionals who are thinking along similar lines, the health care of these people can be rewarding and positive for everyone. Without these essentials, it may seem more like a series of inevitable, overwhelming disasters.

Clinical Exercise

Tackle this case study to see whether you grasp the practicalities of comprehensive geriatric assessment:

Dawn Hill is an 87-year-old woman whose daughters bring her to your family practice office as a new patient. The previous physician didn't seem to be addressing her problems, which (you eventually find) consist of frequently telephoning her two daughters and asking for help.

She lives alone in a small house, takes digoxin 0.25 mg po od, furosemide 40 mg po od, and tolbutamide 500 mg po bid. Her health has been good, except for some heart trouble in the hospital two years ago, diabetes diagnosed by the doctor, and a little bit of recent confusion, according to the daughters. Mrs Hill says she is doing just fine, and glibly denies a functional inquiry.

Bearing in mind that she may be a frail elderly patient, what kind of information would be your next priority:

1. An electrocardiogram, chest x-ray, complete blood count (CBC), electrolytes, glucose, and hemoglobin A1C (turn to 2.1, page 119).

2. A physical examination with focus on ophthalmoscope examination for diabetic retinopathy, jugular venous pressure, lung and precordial auscultation, and ankle edema (turn to 2.2., page 120).

3. A clearer definition of the presenting complaint. What is she calling about? What kind of help is she demanding? Do the daughters agree that there are no specific complaints? (turn to 2.3, page 120).

4. An evaluation of her cognitive performance with one of the mental status questionnaires, a history of her ability to do activities of daily living (confirmed by the family), and a description of what assistance she is receiving at home (turn to 2.4, page 120).

Retinal exam and cardiovascular system are normal, respiratory rate is 20. Your bloodwork (if you chose option 1, above) is normal, with hemoglobin A1C 0.060. Much more to the point, the daughters say Mrs Hill phones each of them 10 to 12 times a day and often makes no sense at all. She repeats herself and does not identify specific problems consistently. Requests include help with the animals (there are none), concern about her husband (he died years ago), and fussing about appointments, which the daughters doubt exist. Although Mrs Hill was eating well, keeping house, dressing appropriately, and staying clean six weeks ago, she now has nothing in the fridge, is evasive about meals, leaves the place in a mess, and has her dress on backwards.

She manages 15/30 on the Folstein Mini-Mental Status Examination, with poor attention to questions.

Within and including a standard medical history, list four or five specific points of subjective information you now require (turn to 2.5, page 121).

After listening to the story, asking penetrating questions, performing a thorough geriatric physical exam, and getting your investigations back, you list the following as Mrs Hill's problems:

Cognitive impairment, probable delirium
Decreased vision
Bilateral cataracts
Ill-fitting dentures
Polypharmacy congestive heart failure medication
Medication noncompliance
Mass left anterior neck
Hyperthyroidism, probable toxic nodular goitre
Status post-cholecystectomy, remote
Status post-appendectomy, remote
Osteoarthritis knees
Mechanical low back pain

Alcohol dependence
Decreased IADL global
Decreased ADL dressing, bathing, and hygiene
Urinary incontinence—no diagnosis
Diabetes, by history
Hypercholesterolemia
Mild liver enzyme elevation

Decide which of these may be remediable and which, if remedied, could significantly improve the recent loss of independence and the confusion, which are Mrs Hill's presenting complaints. Then turn to 2.6, page 121.

CHAPTER 3

Prescribing in the Elderly

Many physicians avoid the frail elderly just because they don't like prescribing for them. This is understandable: complicated elderly people can provide a frustrating and time-consuming clinical challenge in medication management. But these difficulties also eventually deliver the pay-off of reinforcing and teaching us therapeutics, clinical pharmacology, and the joys of common sense in health care.

What makes prescribing for the elderly both difficult and fascinating? The answer is that the outcome is never predictable. The only sure thing about managing medication in old people is that you don't know what's going to happen next. This stimulating situation exists for three important reasons.

First, as people age, they accumulate illness. This means they tend to have a lot of health problems, many of which must be treated with medication. Life is intolerable for a severe Parkinsonian patient off levodopa or for someone in congestive heart failure without a diuretic. The result is that most frail older people take multiple medications, often unavoidably.

Second, the elderly are heterogeneous in the way they handle drugs. As people age, they tend to become more unlike one another in many ways. These include all of the factors that determine response to medication, its dose, and its regimen. Renal function, liver enzyme activity, blood protein, body water and fat, and the way drugs interact with receptor site can be very different across a variety of older individuals. So the plot thickens as we contemplate large numbers of old people (on large numbers of medication), whose responses to the drugs will likely differ from what we expect from reading the pharmacology textbook.

Third, to make matters worse, the elderly take medication variably. Overall, they comply as well as or better than younger people, but the compliance is ill-distributed. Some will take none of their prescribed medication, others all of it, many some days and not others, still others depending on supervision, perceived side effects, recent explanation, the media, and (seemingly) the moon.

Polypharmacy can be defined as inappropriate prescribing. Given the complex starting point, it is easy to see how it might occur. Certain situations can be identified, however, in which wrong prescribing for the elderly regularly arises. Treating symptoms without a diagnosis, which is sometimes possible in single-problemed younger people, leads to too many drugs and the wrong ones in the elderly. Certain drugs are better than others for certain conditions, and in the elderly in general. Pharmacological "concussives," or drugs with a strong effect on the central or autonomic nervous system or on circulation, are poor first choices when others are available. Some drugs, including antidepressants and neuroleptics, which must be given in large doses for young robust individuals, need to be used in tiny quantities in older people.

Finally, polypharmacy arises when there are just too many medications. Using drugs when physical measures might suffice, failing to take advantage of drugs that treat two conditions at once, and not discontinuing medication the indication for which is no longer present can lead to more medication than the patient (or the prescriber) can handle.

We can forgive a physician for wanting to avoid all of this trouble, and we might even wonder a bit about someone who, as a geriatric doctor, actually seeks it out, but reasonable, responsible, by-the-book, and ultimately helpful prescribing for older people is possible. The following rules are guidelines that can serve as starting points. Practice makes perfect; expect the unexpected.

Ten Rules for Prescribing in the Elderly

1. *Don't.* The first rule is to avoid, or at least minimize, all biologically active medicines. This steers us away from polypharmacy, interactions, compliance traps, expense,

and too-difficult questions about which drugs are doing what.

A physical measure may suffice. Heat, ice, massage, transcutaneous electric nerve stimulation (TENS), and stretching replaces non-steroidal anti-inflammatory drugs (NSAIDs) in musculoskeletal conditions; avoiding fluids, timed voiding, underwear pads, and biofeedback may make anticholinergics unnecessary in incontinence.

The other aspect of "don't" is never to use two (or three) drugs when one will do the job. Subspecialist triple therapy for Parkinson's disease, angina, congestive heart failure, or gastroesophageal reflux disease may be efficacious in the abstract, but when all four conditions coexist, the primary care prescriber's common sense is superior by far to the conventional wisdom arising from the double-blind multicentered placebo-controlled trial.

2. *Start low.* Drug doses for the elderly are usually smaller than those for younger adults. Kidneys and liver eliminate medication slower; drugs are distributed through a smaller volume and share less available protein. Therapeutic windows are small. An elderly person may need a full whopping adult dose, but a very small dose may also be toxic.

One fifth to one third of usual starting dose may be appropriate: digoxin 0.0625 mg, hydrochlorothiazide 12.5 mg, diltiazem 30 mg bid, and loxapine 2.5 mg are examples. Even lower doses are occasionally useful. Experiment.

3. *Go slow.* Increase doses slowly, in small increments, allowing extra time for steady state to occur. This is part of the general gingerly, tentative attitude necessary for success. One to two weeks or longer may be safest as a drug's effectiveness is cautiously compared to its possible adverse consequences.

4. *Never start treatment without clear endpoints in mind.* Having decided (sometimes on doubtful evidence) on a trial of medication therapy, it is necessary to begin the exercise in an organized and reasonable way. Recognize that outcome may be beneficial, adverse, neither, or both with each incremental medication change. To act reasonably on returning to evaluate the outcome of a drug prescription or

prescription change, we need to know what we are looking for on the upside and downside.

Will our diuretic cause orthostatic hypotension or incontinence? We will only know for sure if we understand the starting point (did the patient have either problem already?) and if we take the trouble to measure them when we return to evaluate prescription outcome.

5. *Always return to measure the outcome.* Once having prescribed for the elderly routinely, this rule seems so obvious that it shouldn't need to be said, but the most common cause of drug problems in older people may be failure to follow up. In the facility, schedule your next visit to give yourself a fighting chance of taking the next rational step with the drug. At home or in the office, be sure that evaluation of drug prescription outcome is on the agenda for a scheduled visit that occurs reasonably soon.

If elderly response to medication were predictable, this wouldn't matter, but it is anything but predictable, and so it is an absolutely mandatory part of prescribing.

6. *Review the medication at every visit.* Drugs are more often part of the problem than part of the solution in the elderly. Even the briefest and most cursory visit is incomplete without a quick look at what you're up against in the way of polypharmacy. The computer printout in the facility, the pill bottles in plastic bag at the office, the bottles or blister pack at home, and the medication list in the hospital are vital pieces of data. Even if you can remember your own prescribing, beware the consequences of errors, specialists, locums, on-call colleagues, and the patient reaching over the counter.

7. *Risk reducing drugs regularly.* An unnecessary medication is defined as a drug that does not lead to an adverse outcome when reduced or discontinued. Conditions may be temporary, other physicians may have prescribed, and your diagnosis may have been incorrect. The risk-benefit equation may shift once a patient is treated for other conditions. Simplifying the drug routine carries the same pay-off as not prescribing in the first place, and it is part of the regular care of the frail elderly.

Safely reducing a medication is the "mirror image" of safely beginning and gradually increasing it. Having identified a potentially toxic drug, it may be reduced in very small slow increments. The same possibilities exist: adverse outcome (rebound of the condition for which the drug was prescribed), benefit (reduced adverse drug reaction), neither, or both. Returning to measure the outcome of drug reduction is just as important as when prescribing or increasing medication. Conditions that become symptomatic or unstable with drug reduction may be treated with other, less toxic medicines.

8. *One thing at a time.* Titrating medication upward and downward in elderly people can become a complicated confusing business. Ideally, the good and bad consequences of medication changes can be tied to their causes because only one change was being made. This is not always possible, and backtracking and educated guesswork are necessary when in doubt. A slow reduction of medication, for example, may be put on hold while an intercurrent illness is treated and stabilized.

9. *Assure compliance.* Before you can begin making necessary medication changes, you need to be sure the patient is doing (for better or worse) what you intend. Occasionally, this is impossible. Blister packs, other dose-timing devices, supervision, explanation, legible labeling, nonchild-proof lids, and even facility placement may help. An effective compliance enhancer is to follow rule 10.

10. *Keep it simple.* Better compliance, caregiver attention to other tasks, and transparency of interaction and drug outcome reward the tireless pursuit of simple drug regimens. Fortunately, because half-lives are longer in the elderly, once and twice a day scheduling is often possible. Look for "twofers" (treatment of two conditions with one drug): treating angina and hypertension with beta blockers or calcium channel antagonists, congestive heart failure and angina with nitrates, or depression and postherpetic neuralgia with tricyclics are examples.

Other Prescribing Principles

Titrate to ADL. When titrating medication in older people, the good and bad consequences may be hard to keep track of. Fortunately, a final common pathway of benefit and harm from medication (and other treatments) is function, or capacity to perform basic activities of daily living. When in doubt, the drug regimen is optimized when the elderly person is walking best, managing the household capably, or eating independently. Things require further adjustment when these independent functions are collapsing.

Compliance traps. Sudden unexplained problems with medication and their effects may be the result of changes in compliance. Admission to a hospital or facility, visits from out-of-town relatives, a new pharmacist, or worsened symptoms may result in someone's not taking medications according to instructions. Sleep disturbance, delirium due to illness, or addition of a "last straw" new drug may cause compliance to collapse. Review the medication at every visit.

High-yield conditions. Certain conditions are so prevalent among the frail elderly that their treatment and the response to common adverse consequences of the drugs involved are essential elements of a geriatric doctor's repertoire. Depression, Parkinson's disease, agitation in dementia, musculoskeletal pain, and congestive heart failure combined with chronic obstructive lung disease are examples. Caring for frail older people fortunately produces forced familiarity with these problems.

Surveillance. The concept of a stable patient is of little value in frailty. Routine surveillance is necessary because medication regimens, chronic illnesses, and acute problems are always interacting with compliance and social problems to produce unexpected changes. Just when you thought you had a handle on the Parkinson's disease, suspicious behavior arises. A difficult caregiver and problems with finances surface when you least expect them.

Consider cost. Always use the least expensive medicine that may be both effective and safe. Because you are skilled at recognizing subtle adverse drug reactions and good at evaluating benefit, you're in an ideal position to give the best therapeutic bang for the buck.

Clinical Exercise

The following short case study will let you deploy your skills at geriatric therapeutics.

Dal Doperman is a 86-year-old retired musician with congestive heart failure who has just been in the hospital. He was admitted with breathlessness and chest pain, and although he spent three days in the coronary care unit, no final diagnosis for the pain was reached. He was seen by specialists in gastroenterology, rheumatology, respiratory medicine, infectious diseases, and neurology during his stay. A faxed half-page discharge summary handwritten by a resident is illegible. Mr. Doperman's daughter exhibits for you on the breakfast room table pill vials that indicate to you his discharge medications are:

Furosemide 40 mg po od
KCL 600 mg po od
Digoxin 0.25 mg po od
Nifedipine 30 mg "XL" po od
Nitrate slow release 2.6 mg po bid
Sotalol 80 mg po bid
Omeprazole 20 mg po od
Cisapride 10 mg po tid
Amitriptyline 25 mg po at hs
Acetaminophen 325 with codeine 30 mg i po q4h prn pain
Gliclazide 80 mg po bid
Ciprofloxacin 500 mg bid
Clindamycin 150 mg po qid
Enalapril 5 mg po bid
Loxapine 5 mg po tid

The daughter is disturbed that, although her father went into the hospital a pretty sick man, he is now not only much worse than before but worse than he was at his best while in the hospital. He is confused (especially in the evening), very unsteady on his feet, and is losing weight because of a bad appetite. He has constipation and is certainly much less able to look after himself than previously. Although the daughter has three more weeks of holidays, she will be unable to care for him when she returns to work. Social workers at the hospital had suggested a nursing home, but the daughter followed her father's wishes and brought him home instead.

He is pale and thin, attends variably to your questions, manages six out of ten on the Short Portable Mental Status

Questionnaire, has reduced jugular venous pressure, a respiratory rate of 28, reduced air entry but no adventitious sounds in his chest, blood pressure 90/60 sitting, heart rate 50 irregularly irregular, unremarkable abdomen, generalized stiffness and some cogwheel rigidity, and a tentative, slow, stiff, unsafe gait using a cane.

You obtain further collateral history that this man was taking no medication going into the hospital and that he walked well at that time. You call the hospital and a medical records technician reads the following diagnosis from the chart: coronary insufficiency, congestive heart failure, diabetes type II, gastroesophageal reflux disease, dementia with agitation, and pneumonia.

The daughter has been carefully administering his medications for the last four days since discharge.

Pick the likeliest, most-disabling diagnosis from the following list:

1. End-stage heart disease with angina and congestive heart failure (turn to 3.1, page 122).
2. Pneumonia (turn to 3.2, page 122).
3. Parkinson's disease (turn to 3.3, page 122).
4. Multiple drug toxicity (turn to 3.4, page 123).

Assume that Mr. Doperman is having problems caused by medication. You would like to risk reducing or eliminating offending drugs. With which one will you start?

1. Omeprazole (turn to 3.5, page 123).
2. Loxapine (turn to 3.6, page 123).
3. Enalapril (turn to 3.7, page 123).
4. Sotalol (turn to 3.8, page 124).

Geriatrics Topics and Questions

B. Clinical Problems

CHAPTER 4

Mobility Failure

Traditional geriatrics focuses on function and on problems with it, which are referred to as "geriatric giants." One of these is failure of mobility, including falling, unsteadiness, or simply being stuck in a bed or chair. Independence at activities of daily living (ADL) requires, in general, planning and moving around to accomplish tasks. We understand cognitive impairment (see Chapter 6) and recognize it as a major cause of failed ADL. Mobility problems are just as important in failing independence, and one could even characterize frailty as failure of cognition, failure of mobility, or failure of both.

We are practiced at measuring cognition. Mobility measurement is a less precise science, however, and more outcome oriented. As long as you safely get where you're going, the step height, path deviation, speed, and fluidity of motion may not be terribly important. Some of our problems measuring mobility arise because it is studied from diverse points of view by various professionals. Gradually, the study of mobility is crystallizing into a unified understanding of its components, its aging, and the remediable and preventable causes of its failure.

It is still certain that the complicated construct of factors involved in clinical mobility problems requires the knowledgeable efforts of multiple professionals and a lot of time and attention to detail.

Normal Mobility

One can think of staying on one's feet and walking properly as balance (maintaining upright posture), gait (walking and its components), and response to challenges (correcting for trips, pushes, etc.). These three functions involve the entire organism and much of its environment. Position and position-change information arrives at central nervous system coordination structures in the brain (the cerebellum) from vision, mechanoreceptors in the neck, and the semicircular canals in the inner ear. Proprioceptive sensors tell you where the body is at. This automated computer system is controlled by thought through the cerebral cortex and the motor system, which operates through activating muscles, bones, and joints. Problems can arise at any of these stages.

Trouble in maneuvering can also occur because of rushing too quickly, not paying enough attention, being in a dangerous environment, and losing supports (such as lighting or shoes) that one may be accustomed to. Thoughtfulness, attitude, mood, and where one lives can therefore affect mobility.

The biology of gait and balance ages normally, but the whole system can become deconditioned through disuse and can be damaged by illness or injury.

The Specific Mobility Evaluation

When comprehensively assessing a frail old person, or anyone who is falling, unsteady, or unable to walk, a specific gait and balance evaluation needs to be added to your usual repertoire. If there is a "mini-mental status examination" of mobility, it may be the "get up and go" test, now widely used to evaluate gait imbalance.

The patient is seated in an armless chair, 3 m from a wall. He or she stands, walks (with walking aids if usually used) toward the wall, turns without touching the wall, returns to the chair, turns, and sits back down again.

Much more sophisticated and detailed mobility evaluation instruments exist; one can, of course, also evaluate mobility simply by watching someone walk down a hallway. However, the "get up and go" test is a reasonable way to achieve the two broad goals of the gait and balance evaluation: evaluation of safety and data-gathering for diagnosis.

Watching the patient, first ask yourself, How safe does this look? The answer will help in setting up supervision, prescribing walking aids, and possibly restricting free range. Next, look at the pattern of movements to see if any of the remediable causes of mobility failure (see following) are obviously present. Pain, Parkinson's disease, vision problems, unsafe footwear, postural dizziness, and other problems may be more evident here than in the usual physical evaluation.

Remediable Mobility Failure Causes

Two "mega-mnemonics" are presented, one for the mobility failure history and the other for the physical examination. Comprehensive evaluation requires asking the usual functional inquiry questions and doing a standard physical examination. The following lists may help you to run over in your mind the subjective and objective findings that will lead to diagnosing commonly remediable causes of falling, unsteadiness, and failure to ambulate. They are boiled down from a comprehensive list of mobility failure causes, leaving mainly ones amenable to treatment.

CATASTROPHE recalls items on the functional inquiry:

Caregiver and housing
Alcohol (including withdrawal)
Treatment (meaning medications, including compliance)
Affect (presence of depression or lack of initiative)
Syncope (any fainting)
Teetering (dizziness)
Recent illness
Ocular problems
Pain with mobility
Hearing (necessary to avoid hazards)
Environmental hazards

Positive answers on any of these functional inquiry points might direct you to a treatable cause.

When physically evaluating the patient, remember I HATE FALLING to avoid missing any of the following findings:

Inflammation of joints (or deformity)
Hypotension (orthostatic blood pressure change)
Auditory and visual testing
Tremor (or other findings) of Parkinson's disease
Equilibrium (balance) testing
Foot problems
Arrhythmia/block/valve disease in the cardiovascular
   examination
Leg length discrepancy
Lack of conditioning (generalized weakness)
Illness (signs of)
Nutrition poor
Gait disturbance

On a home visit, four items are of particular importance, recalled by CHAT:

Caregiver and housing
Hazards
Alcohol
Taking medications properly?

Recognize that any condition affecting the systems outlined in the preceding description of normal mobility can contribute to mobility failure. These mnemonics and their lists are designed to limit questioning to common remediable problems that will give a high yield in response to treatment. Most mobility failure has several causes. Rarely are all of them remediable, and rarely is any one 100% treatable. Still, a partial influence on a few causes can make a big difference.

Mobility Failure Treatment

The care and treatment of problems with mobility best takes place in a setting of a comprehensive geriatric assessment (see Chapter 2). The first step is to define, list, and try to treat the remediable causes of mobility failure that exist. This can be a complicated and time-consuming process, since treating depression, treating Parkinson's disease, changing medications to improve orthostatic hypotension, intervening with alcohol problems, and obtaining appropriate footwear and walking aids cannot necessarily all be done at once. A plan (with responsibility for each task clearly designated), and some sort of critical path, are very helpful.

Always return to the mobility evaluation ("get up and go" test) to see how you're doing.

The following checklist can help make sure that nothing is missed:

Environmental hazards
Home supports
Socialization and encouragement
Modifying medication
Balance training
Modifying restraints
Involving the family
Facility and homemaker
Follow-up

Once remediable mobility failure causes are identified and tentative treatment started, careful follow-up for possible new problems, adverse consequences of care, and unexpected deterioration can't be over-emphasized.

Controlled trials have suggested that modifying medication and undertaking balance training (usually done by a physiotherapist) are the two items in the preceding list most likely to make a difference in mobility. Common sense may suggest which others are most important in each patient you evaluate.

Clinical Exercise

You are on duty at the hospital emergency room. An 81-year-old man is driven to hospital by his daughters. He has fallen in his first-floor one-bedroom apartment earlier in the day and was unable to get up and call for help. They found him several hours later, conscious but scared and unhappy. He has right hip pain, a forehead laceration, and walks in with assistance.

He says he must have tripped. He was getting lunch (canned beans and a pickle) and went "ass over teakettle" on his way to the fridge. There was no dizziness, vision change, palpitation, or other premonitory symptom. He doesn't think he lost consciousness.

He sees and hears well, doesn't drink, lives alone, and has no pain or weakness in his arms or legs. He takes captopril 12.5 mg po bid and ranitidine 150 mg po bid.

He is alert, oriented, sarcastic, and wants to go home. Physical exam reveals ear wax, decreased air entry in the left chest, regular heart rate of 100, blood pressure 110/70 sitting and standing, a systolic murmur at the apex, a probable abdominal aortic aneurysm, adequate range of movement of both hips, and some corns and calluses. Otherwise, there are no findings. Oral temperature is 35.2°C.

Questions

What is the most common cause of falling in the elderly?

1. Heart block, arrhythmia, or other cause of low cardiac output (turn to 4.1, page 124).
2. Polypharmacy (turn to 4.2, page 124).
3. Multiple causes (turn to 4.3, page 125).
4. Environmental hazards (turn to 4.4, page 125).

You need to generate a working diagnosis here. Which of the usually remediable falling causes might this man have? Turn to 4.5, page 125.

How would you, in an office or emergency room, easily evaluate gait and balance?

1. An in-depth neurological examination (turn to 4.6, page 125).
2. Watch him walking down the hall (turn to 4.7, page 126).
3. The "get up and go test" (turn to 4.8, page 126).

CHAPTER 5

Incontinence

The traditional "geriatric giants" include incontinence, usually taken to mean urinary incontinence, which is a common and distressing symptom in frail older people. The current generation of elderly tend to find matters of elimination unmentionable, which partly explains their embarrassment and reluctance to report incontinence symptoms. Sensitive questioning and an offer of practical assistance is often gratefully welcomed, however.

Disabled older people who don't control urine or bowels may provide professional or family caregivers with a challenge and make life difficult and unpleasant. This is another reason to aggressively seek and treat symptoms of incontinence. It does make a difference to the caregiving dyad.

Incontinence can be a chronic problem due to one or many irremediable causes. On the other hand, recent-onset incontinence may be the result of a single condition or event that is easily correctable. Knowledge of the usual correctable causes and a relatively simple evaluation for their presence is both mandatory and easy.

The definition of *incontinence* depends upon the patient. If it is distressing, the symptom is present and requires evaluation. Distressing would include distressing to the caregiver.

Practical Bladder Physiology

The bladder is a muscular balloon with an outlet held closed by a muscular sphincter. It is emptied by contraction of a detrusor muscle that lies like a cape over the top of the bladder and is innervated by voluntary efferent nerves and

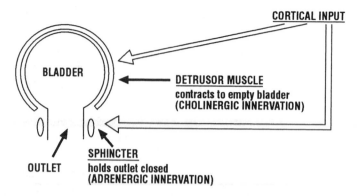

FIGURE 5.1. Functioning of the bladder.

parasympathetic autonomic nervous system neurons from the spinal cord. The sphincter is innervated by adrenergic sympathetic neurons. Urine leaves the bladder via the urethra when bladder pressure exceeds sphincter pressure (see Figure 5.1).

Clinical Classification

Traditionally, urologists and geriatricians have attempted to classify urinary incontinence according to the physiology of its causes and the symptoms usually found in each class. Unfortunately, the more frail the patient, the less clear-cut the clinical picture, and therefore the less useful the classifications become. The most common cause of incontinence in frail people is multiple causes. The history and physical examination may, for once, be of limited value. We present this traditional classification for completeness, however.

Stress incontinence is escape of urine with increased intra-abdominal pressure, usually due to straightening of the urethrovesicle angle as a result of pelvic floor relaxation in females. The history of urine leaking with coughing, bearing down, or laughing may be helpful in older middle-aged patients who could undergo surgery. It is rarely useful in the frail elderly.

Urge incontinence is the common complaint of incontinence shortly after feeling the urge to void, with the need to rush to the toilet. Frequently said to be associated with unstable bladder, this symptom is actually nonspecific as well.

Continuous dribbling incontinence may be due to overflow, with urine leaking from an overfilled bladder in a partial outlet obstruction, or one in which muscle tone is lost (an atonic bladder), where overfilling finally causes the sphincter pressure to be exceeded. Continuous dribbling symptoms are helpful in people who can provide the history, but investigation tends to be the same independent of the pattern of incontinence.

Incontinence Evaluation

Figure 5.2 is an algorithm diagram for evaluation of urinary incontinence. In the algorithm, remediable causes are ruled out in turn. A group of general incontinence causes includes behavioral incontinence (urinating inappropriately to gain attention or annoy caregivers), incontinence due to location (raised bed side rails, distance to the bathroom, or other mobility problems), acute illness from any cause, cognitive function sufficiently impaired to disable the motor planning required to connect a full bladder sensation with making it to the toilet, and finally, medications (diuretics, anticholinergics or any drug that impairs the state of consciousness).

Once these causes are ruled out or treated, evaluation for fecal impaction and a urine culture may turn up two other remediable causes. Asymptomatic bacteriuria is common in the elderly, and it should be corrected once in incontinent patients. If the incontinence persists, the bacteriuria may be assumed to be asymptomatic and can be ignored.

At this point, a urethral catheter should be passed following voiding to determine whether the bladder volume is elevated. If it is greater than 250 ccs, obstruction or atonic bladder is present. If less than 150 ccs, there is probably no significant obstruction or atonic component. From 150 to 250 ccs, some patients benefit from treatment of obstruction, while others do not.

Males with a high post-void residual may have benign prostatic hypertrophy. Finasteride may be very useful in

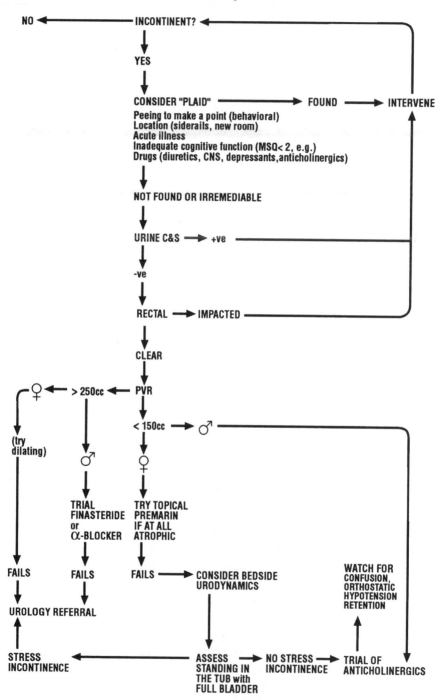

FIGURE 5.2. Incontinence evaluation.

this group of patients, since surgery can be avoided and obstructive incontinence treated indefinitely. Side effects of the drug are few. Alpha-agonists like terazosin may reduce the obstruction-aggravating effect of the sphincter and be temporarily useful. Urology referral may be necessary for investigation and correction of outlet obstruction. An atonic bladder most often follows an obstructive episode. Catheterization (sometimes for many weeks) may be necessary to reestablish voiding. Bethanachol is occasionally useful.

Females with known benign stricture may be dilated under local anaesthetic in the office or long-term care facility. Otherwise, urology referral for dilatation or investigation is necessary. Low post-void residual females may respond to topical or systemic estrogens if atrophic urethritis is a significant cause. A trial of therapy is usually helpful.

If stress incontinence seems a real possibility, suprapubic bladder suspension or other surgical procedures may be considered. Urodynamics may be helpful to rule out unstable bladder, which may make surgery pointless.

Males with low post-void residual and no other remediable causes and females in whom the aforementioned causes have been ruled out often have unstable bladders (*detrusor instability* and *bladder dyssynergy* are synonyms). Drugs for this condition, in which the detrusor muscle contracts in an uncontrolled way, include oxybutinin, propantheline, and other anticholinergics. Flavoxate, nifedipine, and imipramine have been tried with occasional success as well. Careful attention to side effects of confusion and orthostatic hypotension are mandatory. Start low, go slow.

Occasionally, patients respond to adrenergic agonists (eg, pseudoephedrine) or beta blockers if a lax or overly vigorous sphincter are the problem. Trials of therapy will help to sort these cases out, avoiding the need for expensive and often futile urodynamics.

Nondrug treatment using timed voiding, biofeedback, and other bladder training systems may be helpful, either in conjunction with drugs or alone.

Catheterization for incontinence is a treatment of last resort, occasionally useful temporarily in skin breakdown.

Better are "containment systems," diapers that allow a semblance of normal activity. These are extensively used in extended-care facilities.

Ruling out remediable causes and careful trials of therapy (recognizing the risk of toxicity) is the usual activity in caring for incontinent patients. Remember that the most common cause is multiple causes and that the situation may change.

Clinical Exercises

Case 1

Yuri Blokov is a 75-year-old man living in extended care who has been incontinent for a long and indeterminate time. You assume his care and wonder about remediability. He is nonambulatory since a left parietal infarct five years ago, with right hemiplegia, global aphasia, and probably some cognitive impairment. The incontinence is constant, worse when he first is taken out of bed in the morning. He requires incontinence briefs at all times.

This man needs one person for transfer to bed from chair, is cooperative with dressing and bathing, and feeds himself with his left hand.

He takes no medicine except enteric-coated acetylsalicylic acid (ASA) 325 mg i po od and has no evidence of an acute illness. Cognitively, he is difficult to measure because of the communication problems.

What might be your first step in dealing with this problem?

1. Start a trial of oxybutinin to see if he responds (turn to 5.1, page 126).
2. Catheterize him in and out to determine whether he is obstructed (turn to 5.2, page 126).
3. Check for fecal impaction and urinary tract infection (turn to 5.3, page 127).
4. This man is too impaired to be continent in any case: incontinence briefs are your only option (turn to 5.4, page 127).

Case 2

Cecile Faireau, an 80-year-old woman living alone in an apartment, presents in your office with a complaint of incontinence. She describes losing her urine, gradually worsening over several months, in various circumstances. After feeling the urge to void (and although she walks well), she must hurry to reach a toilet, otherwise urine leaks. There is some leakage with laughing and coughing, and she does find some problems at night.

She has no dysuria, no hesitancy, no history of genitourinary surgery, takes no medications, and is completely well otherwise.

Urine culture is positive for 100,000 colonies *E. coli*; post-void residual (PVR) 25 cc.

You treat her urinary tract infection (UTI) successfully, and there is no change in the symptom. What now?

1. A trial of therapy with flavoxate 200 mg po tid (turn to 5.5, page 127).
2. Recommend timed frequent toileting (turn to 5.6, page 127).
3. A trial of topical estrogen (turn to 5.7, page 127).
4. Referral to urology or gynecology for a bladder suspension procedure (turn to 5.8, page 128).

CHAPTER 6

Cognitive Impairment

Aging entails, among other things, loss of physiological reserve. Young organ systems function with plenty of extra capacity; older ones are less elastic, and their ability to compensate for stress may be exceeded. The more complicated the system or function, the more sensitive it may be. So it is with the aging brain.

Geriatric physicians think of higher mental function like that of any other organ system and encounter its failure routinely. We recognize (by analogy to respiratory failure or renal failure) two syndromes of brain failure: one acute, one chronic.

Delirium is the acute organic brain syndrome in which a physical insult to an aging brain causes acute failure of its higher function. *Dementia* is the chronic organic brain syndrome in which a particular illness or injury causes permanent damage. As with the lungs or kidneys, one often sees chronic failure with superimposed acute injury, that is, both syndromes at once.

In the past, reversible cognitive impairment was thought to be fairly common. Unfortunately, it is less so than we used to believe, even when the problem is true pure delirium. Still, no matter how irreversible brain damage may be, its impact can be minimized by good medical and social care, which allow existing strengths to be most usefully manifested.

Confusion Triage

Patients presenting or presented as confused may be cognitively impaired. A system for beginning their evaluation is presented in Figure 6.1. Standard instruments to measure memory, orientation, calculation, attention, and other higher mental functions are used to evaluate the patient. If impairment of these functions (cognitive impairment) exists, it can be roughly quantified by instruments such as the Folstein Mini-mental Status Examination, the Short Portable Mental Status Questionnaire, and the 3MS.

Confronted with definite or suspected cognitive impairment, as indicated by poor performance on the aforementioned tests, the next step in evaluating confusion is to rule out the presence of delirium. If delirium is not present, a tentative diagnosis of dementia may be made by exclusion. If delirium is present, its reversible causes must be sought. Difficulty with attention, indicating possible delirium, exists when someone is unable to follow a pattern of calculation or to repeat numbers in reverse out of proportion with the amount of overall cognitive impairment already found. Someone scoring 7 or 8 on the Folstein Mini-mental Status Examination would not be expected to calculate, because of

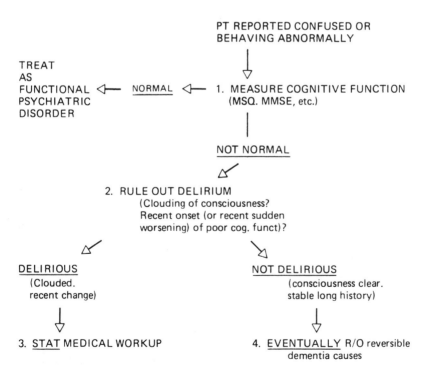

FIGURE 6.1. Confusion triage.

advanced dementia. Someone scoring between 22 and 25, however, should be able to attend to simple calculation tasks. Clouding of the state of consciousness, manifested as a drunken or distractible type of behavior, is another hint that delirium may be present. Patients sick with fever, hospitalized with surgical illness, or otherwise in a setting of unstable health raise a high index of suspicion for delirium.

The most challenging confusion triage is the moderately or severely demented patient who undergoes an apparent acute change in cognition. Is there delirium, is its cause reversible, and will it influence management?

Delirium

The *Fourth Diagnostic and Statistical Manual of Psychiatry* (DSM IV) defines *delirium* as loss of attention and changes in consciousness. There must also be cognitive change or impairment, or disturbance of perception, and a short and fluctuating time course. One must then specify the causes of delirium to complete the DSM IV classification.

It is a basic principle of geriatrics that the delirious patient requires prompt and thorough medical evaluation. Although many delirium states remain undiagnosed after our best efforts, many more are the result of simple must-treat conditions, which can be serious or dangerous.

A simple mnemonic (CAMP squared) assists in remembering the most common and easily treated delirium causes. Central nervous system (CNS) disease (stroke, subdural hematoma, or other acute brain condition) indicates the group of gross brain disease causing focal neurological findings, which may be visible on a CT scan of the head. Congestive heart failure may be atypical and present simply with state-of-consciousness changes. Alcohol intoxication or withdrawal and all the causes of the traditional surgical acute abdomen are two other causes. Metabolic causes include virtually all conditions easily identifiable with a blood test. High or low blood levels of sodium, glucose, potassium, calcium, magnesium, etc.; hyper and hypo function of the thyroid or adrenals (or other glands); and renal or hepatic system failure are broadly in this group. Medication of any kind may be a cause of delirium, especially sedative, anticholinergic, or hypotension-causing medication. Pyrexia includes respiratory, urinary, intra-abdominal, and CNS infections, and "psychological" reminds that some apparent delirium is really an Axis I psychiatric disorder.

While the causes of delirium are searched for, the patient requires careful symptomatic treatment, with reassurance (including that of the relatives and caregivers), a darkened and quiet environment without sudden changes or unfamiliar activity, and the careful and frequently reevaluated use of benzodiazepines or neuroleptic medication to obtain cooperation, prevent injury, and relieve psychological distress.

Dementia

The DSM IV defines dementia simply as a cognitive deficit, resulting in memory impairment, some neurobehavioral component (aphasia, apraxia, agnosia, or decreased executive function), accompanied by a significant decrease in social function, and by criteria specific to the various dementia causes.

Alzheimer's disease usually pursues a gradually progressive course, with neurobehavioral problems and memory deficit early in the disease. Vascular (formerly multiple infarct) dementia results in a neuropsychologically "spotty" picture, with defects on the Folstein Mini-Mental Status Examination that are not global and often in focal neurological findings as well as evidence of damage due to atherosclerosis elsewhere.

Dementia due to trauma carries a history of injuries and may also have focal neurological findings associated. "Substance-induced persisting" dementia is most commonly due to alcohol. Other chronic alcohol-related syndromes, such as Wernecke's encephalopathy or amnestic syndrome, may also be present.

Specific features of Huntington's or Parkinson's disease may be present. A very common dementia cause is two or more of the above: mixed dementia. Recently, a syndrome of loss of judgment, disinhibition, hypersexuality, and other symptoms of loss of social function as early findings in dementia are classed as frontoparietal dementias. Testing for these is evolving; treatment is of course well in the future.

A famous mnemonic (DEMENTIA) indicates a list of "reversible" causes of dementia, but it is actually mainly useful in identifying co-morbidity in cognitively impaired people. Drugs, emotional problems (depression), metabolic problems (see delirium above), eyes and ears (deafness and blindness), nutritional/neurological (B12 and other vitamin deficiencies and gross lesions in the CNS), tumors and trauma, infection (including syphilis, infective endocarditis, and HIV), and atherosclerosis, alcohol, and anemia, is the list this mnemonic brings to mind.

In practical terms, profound hypothyroidism, subdural hematoma, normal pressure hydrocephalus, a slow-growing meningioma, drug toxicity, and severe depression is a more useful list to recall as a starting point for ruling out reversible dementia causes. Sadly, these causes often either have resulted in irremediable damage or co-exist with a more common irreversible dementia cause, and so result in little improvement when treated.

Alzheimer's disease treatment is notoriously unsuccessful. Numerous drugs have been claimed to be effective, but none truly reverses or cures the illness. Tacrine appears in clinical trials to improve functional capacity in relatively advanced dementia. Good comprehensive geriatric evaluation may turn up several remediable conditions that, when treated, give at least the impression of improvement in dementia severity.

If avoiding institutionalization is a desired outcome in dementia care, support given to informal caregivers seems to be the most consistently successful intervention. Treatment of disturbing and occasionally dangerous psychological symptoms with drugs is a real challenge and requires our best geriatric prescribing behavior (see Chapter 3). Depression and agitation are the two most frequently encountered symptoms. These subjects are treated in Chapters 7 and 10, respectively.

Neuropsychologists are skilled at measuring specific cognitive abilities and impairments. For those of us amateurs who must evaluate cognition without their in-depth training, certain shortcuts are available. The Folstein Mini-Mental Status Examination and Short Portable Mental Status Questionnaire do provide numeric scores that very roughly correspond to severity of cognitive impairment. They are also fairly reproducible among various professionals and within the same patient. Unfortunately, many patients who score well on these tests are intelligent people with compensatory mechanisms that may hide significant dementia. Others who do poorly may be merely culturally different, anxious, lacking in intelligence, hearing-impaired, or not interested in the process. Temper simple cognitive measurement with common sense and a view to the global picture.

The 3MS is a longer, more demonstrably reproducible, and more sensitive evaluation instrument now used increasingly. It includes evaluation of skills such as naming similarities between pairs of objects, and generating lists of classes of objects (eg, four-legged animals). Its length and complexity may be justified, depending on the circumstances.

Delirium must be tested in context as well. Serial subtraction and digit span are valuable tests, but a setting of illness and the high index of suspicion that should accompany this testing is at least as useful in identifying cases of delirium.

Clinical Exercise

An 84-year-old Asian gentleman is in your community acute care hospital, and nursing calls at 0130 to request your evaluation (as nighttime physician on call) of an acute deterioration.

Reading the chart, you are frustrated but not surprised to find very limited past medical history, no record of cognitive function prior to admission, no notation of living circumstances or level of independence prior to admission, and an extremely succinct operating room report of surgery about 36 hours ago, which appears to say "right hemicolectomy."

Nursing states that the man is confused. He has tried to climb out of bed and has pulled out his intravenous line. Shouting has disturbed other patients, and a sedative is requested.

Current medications include nifedipine 60 mg "XL" po od, furosemide 40 mg po od, finasteride 5 mg po od, morphine 1–2 mg IV q1h prn pain, and cefuroxime 500 mg IV q12h.

The man looks frightened, is cool and dry, appears pale and thin, and has no visible neck veins. Blood pressure is 90/60 lying flat, respiratory rate 28, audible heart sounds, and a silent, tender abdomen with a recent, clean surgical scar.

Focusing on the presentation of confusion, what is the first thing you wish to establish?

1. Is he cognitively impaired? (Turn to 6.1, page 128.)
2. Does he have a psychiatric history? (Turn to 6.2, page 128.)
3. Is the problem entirely one of language? (Turn to 6.3, page 128.)
4. Is he septic? (Turn to 6.4, page 129.)

Through a nurse fluent in Cantonese you discover the following: he knows the name of your city and that he is in the hospital, but he does not recall the operation. He knows the month, misses the date by 10 days, and gives you an incorrect year. He recalls two of three objects after distraction, but he is unwilling or unable to do arithmetic or spell forward or backwards. He complains of abdominal pain and says that otherwise he feels fine.

What is going on at this stage?

1. He is cognitively impaired but not delirious (turn to 6.5, page 129).
2. He is cognitively intact, allowing for language (turn to 6.6, page 129).
3. He is delirious, so cognitive performance cannot be evaluated (turn to 6.7, page 130).

4. He is cognitively impaired, and delirium cannot be ruled in or out from the information available so far (turn to 6.8, page 130).

Testing his digit span indicates a state of attention appropriate and expected for his level of cognitive impairment. You contact his family physician, and discover that he is often hypotensive (he takes the nifedipine for angina), he has chronic obstructive lung disease and is breathless at rest, and that he has had gradually accumulating Alzheimer's disease for about three years. Blood work, including oxygen saturation, chest x-ray, and abdominal films are negative, and you prescribe a once-only benzodiazepine as treatment for your working diagnosis of relocation stress in dementia. He recovers uneventfully and returns to his intermediate care nursing home.

CHAPTER 7

Depression

Serious disabling unhappiness and aging both carry negative meanings for many people, the former legitimately, the latter with no real justification. Granted, depression is common in the elderly; losses often accompany aging, and despondency may be the only response left for someone with no assets who is overwhelmed by a popular expectation of misery. Elderly men, for some reason, are especially vulnerable to the illness we know as depression. Suicide rates increase linearly with age. Is this all to some extent a self-fulfilling expectation?

Just identifying depressed elderly people is challenging. Several chronic physical illnesses can produce symptoms similar to those of depression and may cause depression itself. Medication is often a cause of secondary depression and can produce depression-like states. Loss of cognitive ability, in its early stages, can be depressing, and depression can lead to poor performance at testing in someone cognitively completely normal.

Normal aging is a complex psychological and social experience. It may include sleep and dietary changes, slowing down of activity, and a less enthusiastic response to pleasures considered essential in younger adults. If one expects getting old to be dreadful, there may be little basis for developing habits of joy and satisfaction in later years. Many elderly people with depressive illness are simply considered normally and justifiably sour about an unavoidable fate.

We use criteria for mood disorder diagnosis that have not been validated in the elderly. They may never be, because psychological and biological heterogeneity in this age group makes it hard to strike criteria both inclusive and specific.

The diagnosis, therefore, is often suspected rather than confirmed by a descriptive formula, and a cautious trial of biological treatment may be the only or the best test for the presence of the disease.

DSM Terminology

The Diagnostic and Statistical Manual of Psychiatry (DSM IV) is highly validated and widely accepted. Although its descriptions may be blurred in a heterogeneous elderly population, physicians caring for depressed elderly people should understand its terminology and criteria as a first-order basis for diagnosis.

A major depressive episode (MDE) consists of two weeks of any five of the famous nine criteria, which should probably be on everyone's list of memorizables. Either dysphoria or anhedonia must be present, and then any four others, including weight or appetite change, sleep disturbance, psychomotor rate change, fatigue or loss of energy, guilt or feelings of worthlessness, poor concentration or indecisiveness, and a suicide attempt or ideation or thoughts of death. MDE by these criteria is consistent with depression in the elderly, but beware of atypical presentations of any of the criteria, false positives due to normal aging changes, and false negatives when the history is difficult to obtain.

Major depressive disorder (MDD) is the diagnosis when MDE is present, not due to another illness, and without mania.

An unhappy elderly person may be suffering from dysthymia if there is a two-year history of depressed mood that does not amount to MDE. Simple bereavement and adjustment disorder (depressed mood) mean that a state of unhappiness exists that we can clearly connect to a major negative event. When cognitive impairment is definitely present and memory impairment, disorientation, and failure at activities requiring thought are more important parts of the problem than unhappiness itself, the primary diagnosis may be dementia. Depression can co-exist with dementia or be secondary to it.

Morbid grief is a state of unhappiness in response to tragic life events. It is not mentioned in the DSM, but it occurs in the elderly and can appear as depression.

Many unhappy older persons fit neatly into DSM categories and can be cared for based on this classification. It is, however, only a starting point, and trials of therapy, periods of observation, and second opinions may be necessary to reach the most useful diagnostic formulation and treatment strategies.

Secondary Depression

Because chronic painful conditions and the use of multiple medications are seen frequently in older people, depression as a result of physical illness or as a drug effect is also quite common. The advantage of identifying this secondary depression is that it can be successfully treated if the underlying cause can be modified. Usual depression treatment with psychotherapy, drugs, and electroconvulsive therapy (ECT) is not likely to be successful if the depression is secondary, unless the cause is treated, too.

Any medication can contribute to depression, but certain drugs are frequent offenders. Beta blockers, alpha-methyldopa, reserpine (and other older antihypertensives), narcotics, NSAIDs, L-dopa, all sedatives, and corticosteroids are drugs worth considering as possible secondary depression causes. Alcohol dependence or abuse is a frequent (and frequently hidden) cause as well. Alcohol trouble can be secondary to depression, a vicious cycle requiring careful chicken-and-egg evaluation.

Any major medical condition can create a state of chronic unhappiness indistinguishable from depression. Most potently, painful conditions such as any arthritis, post-herpetic neuralgia, and cancer interrupt pleasure and emphasize unhappiness. Parkinson's disease and stroke are frequent accelerators of depression.

If a secondary depression cause is suspected, treating it as thoroughly as possible is a good first approach to the mood disorder. Antidepressants may be necessary and may help, later on, but go for the cause, if you can find one.

Atypical Presentation of Depression

As we discussed earlier in the section on DSM terminology, textbook depressive features may be present in some elderly patients. Although a purist may insist that the classic criteria always exist in some subtle, hidden form, a majority of depressed elderly seem to show only non-textbook manifestations. Lots of apparently irremediable physical complaints shifting from system to system may be the tip of a depressive iceberg. Heavy alcohol drinking that appears newly in an older person or a change in behavior emphasizing social isolation and withdrawal from family activities are often indications of depression. A cognitively impaired person who becomes agitated and persistently importuning may be depressed. Self neglect or the "geriatric failure to thrive" syndrome (dwindling or deteriorating ADL ability without a clear explanation) may respond to depression treatment. "Depression equivalent" means pain or other physical symptoms with non-organic features that disappear when a mood disorder is controlled.

Depression is similar to many conditions in challenging us with atypical presentations. It should come to mind (along with medication effects) in any situation where an elderly person is having problems that defy usual diagnostic and treatment strategies.

Depression and Cognition

Cognitive impairment (see Chapter 6) is common in frail older people, as is depression. The two conditions may, of course, co-exist. Unlike most cognitive impairment, mood disorder responds to treatment and should therefore be suspected and treated in unhappy patients with dementia.

Once effective treatment is in place, the mood will improve, and any portion of the apparent cognitive impairment that was due to depression will disappear as well. Most likely, the response (if any) will be mood improvement alone.

Treatment of Depression

MDD in the elderly usually requires biological treatment (drugs or ECT), as well as psychotherapy and caregiver support. Psychotherapy alone is rarely effective.

Drug treatment of depression is no exception to the principles of prescribing outlined in Chapter 3. Some adverse consequences will offset any benefit, and your tireless repeated evaluation of the consequences of drug treatment is absolutely mandatory.

We find that excellent geriatric psychiatry experts currently differ on "first choice" drug treatment of depression in the elderly. Generally, selective serotonin reuptake inhibitors (SSRIs) are now first-line treatment in mild to moderate depression because of their relatively benign side-effect profile. They may cause weight loss and agitation in the early stages of treatment, and low doses, careful monitoring, and long (sometimes extremely long) trial periods are necessary. Currently four SSRIs are available (fluoxetine, fluvoxamine, sertraline, and paroxetine). Each drug may be effective and relatively free of side effects even when others have been ruled out. Fluoxetine has an unacceptably long half life for most frail elderly. Paroxetine and fluoxetine interfere with liver enzymes and produce unpredictable changes in other drugs. Sertraline may increase the effect of warfarin.

Moclobemide is a selective monoamine oxidase inhibitor, which is used more and more frequently in MDD and in depression associated with Parkinson's disease. It must be used in adequate doses, and it seems to cause few adverse drug reactions.

Among tricyclic antidepressants, nortriptyline and desipramine have long been favored for elderly patients. Both drugs have autonomic effects. Orthostatic hypotension and delirium are possible but may be avoided by "starting low and going slow." Many experts believe that nortriptyline is preferable to SSRIs in severe depression. Low blood level lithium, or L-thyroxine may be added to potentiate tricyclic antidepressants. An SSRI can be added to nortriptyline or another tricyclic antidepressant if side effects prohibit adequate doses of the latter. Venlafaxine may combine the benefits of SSRIs and tricyclics.

Electroconvulsive therapy, still victim of bad popular press, is excellent treatment for depression in older people who do not tolerate or respond to medication. Some severe and extremely neurovegetatively dense depression requires ECT at the outset. Occasionally, "maintenance" ECT is necessary, and an older person may be brought to the hospital every few months for repeat treatments.

Depression is a must-diagnose and must-treat condition in the frail elderly. Its morbidity and suffering are extreme, although often hidden, and its treatment generally effective. Suspect it often, and treat it carefully and effectively.

Clinical Exercise

78-year-old Dolores Down is referred to your geriatric day hospital because of failure of independence. Six months ago, she was maintaining her apartment with home-support help, doing her own simple banking, taking the bus, and participating with her daughter in weekly shopping. She heated meals and attended a bridge club. Now, she goes out less, isn't eating as well, has lost some weight, and isn't keeping up her end of the house cleaning. Bills are unpaid, and she has quit playing cards.

Always otherwise well, Dolores has had cholecystectomy, hysterectomy, fracture of the right hip, and hypertension, but has taken them in her stride.

Her husband died 10 years ago, and her grief was severe but short-lived. She takes hydrochlorothiazide 25 mg po once daily, and propranolol 40 mg po bid for high blood pressure. She does smoke, and takes a drink of whiskey every night with her dinner.

Your functional inquiry, when you see her, elicits a lot of complaints spanning virtually every system. She scores 28 of 30 on Folstein Mini-Mental Status Examination, missing the floor location of your unit, and crumples the paper instead of handing it back to you. "Leave me alone" is her sentence. She denies being depressed, except by the failure of her health, but she cannot identify a truly pleasurable activity. Her energy is poor, she sleeps well, denies guilt or trouble concentrating, is shocked at the mention of suicide, and her psychomotor rate may be somewhat slowed.

Your physical examination is normal for her age, except for a symptomatic orthostatic blood pressure drop.

Considering the usual criteria, is Mrs. Down having a major depressive episode?

1. Yes, she does fulfill DSM-IV criteria (turn to 7.1, page 130).
2. No, she doesn't fulfill DSM-IV criteria (turn to 7.2, page 131).
3. DSM-IV criteria and diagnostic labels are irrelevant here; she is obviously depressed (turn to 7.3, page 131).
4. The propranolol is probably causing her mood problems, so this is secondary depression, not MDE (turn to 7.4, page 131).

You accept that the working diagnosis is depression and decide to pursue both a biological and psychological treatment strategy.

While she is in enrolled in a socialization program, choose from the following list the antidepressant medication regime you would start:

1. Venlafaxine 75 mg po once daily (turn to 7.5, page 131).
2. Sertraline 50 mg po once daily (turn to 7.6, page 132).
3. Fluoxetine 10 mg po once daily (turn to 7.7, page 132).
4. Nortryptiline 10 mg po once daily (turn to 7.8, page 132).

CHAPTER 8

Abuse, Alcohol, and Automobiles

Social problems that arise from conflict between people, from substance abuse, and from safety hazards can disrupt any stage of life. Elderly people are no exception, and yet they may fall more catastrophically victim to some of these difficulties. As with other aspects of health and illness, the special problems older people encounter here involve frailty, and the disability and vulnerability that accompany it. Like illness, many social difficulties do not present themselves to us as readily and as neatly as they do in younger, "typical" patients.

In this chapter, we consider three common problems encountered in caring for aging people that may challenge us and require an organized approach: elder abuse, substance abuse (particularly alcohol), and motor vehicle driving safety.

Elder Abuse

Recently we have recognized physical, emotional, sexual, nutritional, or financial advantage-taking of older people as surprisingly common. Elderly victims are often helpless to protect themselves against or to object to treatment that would raise howls of protest (and result in prompt punishment) if directed at a younger victim.

Simply leaving an elderly person without adequate support and care can result in his or her psychological or physical injury, and so we may think of abuse as being passive (neglect) or active.

There is no "typical" abused elder. Statistically, however, certain groups emerge as likely victims, producing a composite of the most-abused person. A physically dependent female who controls the finances or directs other important aspects of another person's life may attract abuse. If the person has a problem that a caregiver finds difficult (incontinence, agitated behavior, wandering, or persistent pain), the problem is compounded. An abusive person may see cognitive impairment as a barrier to the victim's reporting abuse.

Caregivers who are alone and suffer a severe burden of care, those financially dependent on an older person who in turn depends on them for care, difficult or aggressive individuals, and substance abusers (particularly people who abuse alcohol) are statistically more likely to be abusive than others who do not share these characteristics.

One can discern common sense in these profiles of abused and abuser; they are also merely guidelines, and exceptions abound; abuse happens among the nicest people.

When you suspect abuse, and as a matter of routine, look for evidence of injury in frail older people. Unusual injuries (breast or genital, improbable fractures) are suspicious. Weight loss has many causes, but absence of an organic or psychological reason in a setting where a caregiver would normally provide food suggests neglect. Deterioration in activities of daily living without explanation (the geriatric failure to thrive syndrome) may be due to abuse. Patients in potentially harmful situations who exhibit poor hygiene of body or clothing merit extra attention. Any of these characteristics may seem to be a consequence of aging, cognitive impairment, or poverty.

There is often a co-dependency, with consequent fear of reprisal and abandonment. An old person who is helpless in terms of activities of daily living (ADL) may withstand abuse as though it were a price to be paid for caregiving. Look discretely at every caregiver relationship with a skeptical raised eyebrow at least once.

If abuse is suspected, the safety of the older person must first be assured. Removing him or her from the situation, or confronting or arresting a perpetrator may be necessary if good judgment indicates a real danger. At this point, assistance with caregiving must be provided, sometimes urgently. Try to find alternatives to hospital admission.

But more often, an abusive situation is mixed with one in which valuable caregiving is provided. The challenge here is not to destroy the beneficial side of the arrangement. Counseling and supervision may uncover remediable reasons for the difficulty, and surveillance with help and respite may do the trick. An obvious open-and-shut situation is usually the tip of a surprising iceberg.

Alcohol

Stability in frailty may rest on numerous shaky pillars of support. Lowly alcohol may be one of these, and dependence upon it or frank substance abuse may be all that stands between a fragile older person and collapse into facility, hospital, or despair. The dangers of alcohol toxicity, intoxication, withdrawal, and its medical consequences are magnified, however, by aging, and treatment is both more necessary and more difficult than it is in younger people.

Detecting alcohol dependence or abuse in older people is difficult. Geriatric giants may be the presentation. Hospitalized patients or newly placed facility residents may present with a non-textbook withdrawal syndrome. A suicide attempt may mean that alcohol has led to depression or that it has recently failed as a last resort.

The CAGE questionnaire is useful for screening, but negative answers must be viewed with suspicion if other indications are present. Morning drinking ("eye-openers") obviously is a graver sign than failed attempts to cut down, annoyance at attention paid to the habit, or guilt.

Older people who drink excessively may be classified as late starters: perhaps they were "social" drinkers in early life who are accelerating due to retirement or relationship changes; outliers among alcoholics who somehow survived the minefield of GI hemorrhages, motor vehicle accidents, cardiomyopathy, and psychosocial disaster; and symptomatic drinkers who are escaping from depression or pain of chronic disease.

The social opprobrium of alcohol is often a huge obstacle in the present generation of elderly. People practicing heavy drinking denied it during their youth even more often than they do today, and many apparently failing elderly people will hide their problem (or that of their spouse) to the bitter end.

Unlike younger substance abusers, a 180-degree turnaround into abstinence is often simply not possible. Elderly people who rely on alcohol for symptom control, psychological stability, or freedom from withdrawal symptoms may not be able to maintain an already unstable independence if they are forced to stop suddenly.

As a caregiver, developing a trust and rapport helps in controlling the problem for the elderly patient, so that it can be minimized without abrupt changes and irreversible collapses. Understanding and sympathy may provide reassurance that abrupt changes will not occur, and they may win trust. This is an area where it is worth spending some valuable time.

Confrontating an elderly denying drinker is rarely productive. Often, however, negative symptoms can be tied to the alcohol habit in a productive way to encourage reduced intake. Tremor, cognitive impairment, depression in withdrawal, abdominal pain, medication problems, falls, social isolation, and sleep disturbance are all troublesome to rational older people. Convincing them that alcohol abuse contributes to or causes these difficulties may be a worthwhile first step.

However the problem is addressed, it is no less chronic than osteoarthritis or chronic obstructive lung disease. Frequent visits, continued reassurance, control of intake short of abstinence, symptom relief, and treatment of other frailty-producing conditions are an ongoing challenge.

Driving

Elderly drivers can make up in experience something of what they lack in reaction time and reduced hearing and vision. Hopefully, that experience teaches that caution must increase as the changes of aging begin to blunt capability at what is sometimes a very demanding activity.

For a caregiver or custodian of public safety, any danger an elderly person behind the wheel may pose on the road must be carefully weighed against the great benefit of independence that car driving provides. If real problems with driving exist, then instrumental activities of daily living, which include banking, shopping, visiting friends, or running a small business, must be watched carefully, and driving minimized, especially in terms of high-ways, nighttime, and rush-hour exposure. Assistance with replacing the automobile as a means of getting around and expressing one's independence and individuality must be provided.

Motor vehicle accidents are relatively random events and difficult to study statistically. Studies and common sense assist us in recognizing the health problems that can in-crease the risk of a crash. Seizures are pretty well an absolute contraindication to driving, although control for one year and good medication compliance may reverse this. Cardiac arrhythmia is dangerous only if symptomatic, angina only if unstable, and arthritis only if it impairs turning to look over the shoulder and the ability to move the extremities quickly enough to steer and operate the pedals. Parkinson's disease is a problem in proportion to bradykinesia and rigidity; tremor alone does not usually impair safety. Diabetics are dangerous only if true hypoglycemic episodes can occur. Problem drinkers should always be off the road until the problem is convinc-ingly solved. The use of sedative, insulin, and antide-pressant medication may create somnolence or other disturbances of consciousness, which are a problem in driv-ing Finally, you have to see to drive, and visual testing is necessary.

Dementia and driving needs consideration, separately from the aforementioned health problems. Cognitively im-paired people, especially Alzheimer's patients, may have good vision and excellent motor function. Their difficulty, however, is with planning and organizing complex tasks. Certain traffic situations may be dangerous to people whose eyesight and reaction times are very good, if they are un-able to register multiple pieces of information, decide and execute sequential actions, or remember where they are going. Recognizing the limitations of instruments and scores, a score of less than 22 on the Folstein Mini-mental Status Examination should alert an evaluator that these functions may be impaired. A score of less than 16, all other things being equal, likely indicates danger on the road.

Riding in a car with a demented person can be a revealing experience. If in doubt about ability, take a ride in varied traffic situations and ask yourself how safe you feel. If your sixth sense tells you you'd prefer to be in an armored car, trust it. Evaluate the driver's judgment in discretionary situations. Remember that progressive dementia will lead to limitation of independence sooner rather than later, and plan for IADL support, rather than allowing a doubtful driver to create a hazard.

Clinical Exercise

Case 1

Cible Beaton, age 88, lives in a large frame house with her single son. She has severe osteoarthritis, with failed hip prostheses bilaterally, and symptomatic knees. She is cognitively intact, but her mobility is further impaired by having had lacunar strokes, which affect coordination and balance. She takes no medication but does require full support for instrumuntal activities of daily living (IADL). She is chairfast.

Her son assists with transfers and toileting at night and on weekends. Daytime (while he works), a full-time home-maker is present.

On your routine three-monthly home visit, the patient complains of pain in her shoulders, which is new. Physical examination shows a very marked reduced range of movement in abduction bilaterally, which you don't recall from before. Mrs. Beaton also looks thin, and weighing her discloses a 5 kg weight loss in three months. During routine questioning, she volunteers that her son is drinking, and that he has been "a bit rough" with her at times. He has also reduced the home support worker's visits to two days per week, leaving the patient alone many days. She becomes tearful in describing her frustration, since they cannot afford full-time caregivers. She is guilty about her influence over the son, whose income is low and who expects to inherit the house. It is clear she fears living with him but is at the same time determined not to enter a facility.

What next?

1. Immediately contact the community authorities and report this abusive situation (turn to 8.1, page 132).
2. Telephone the son and request that he drop in to your office for an appointment to discuss his mother's health (turn to 8.2, page 133).
3. Reassure Mrs. Beaton that things will probably settle down, and suggest that she be friendly and conciliatory toward her son, while waiting to see what happens (turn to 8.3, page 133).
4. Recommend to the patient that she contact a psychologist skilled at counseling elderly (turn to 8.4, page 133).

Case 2

Olive Martini, age 76, has admitted to a home care nurse that she has a drinking problem. The nurse (sworn to secrecy) promptly calls and tells you, confirming your suspicion of several years. Mrs. Martini has mild cognitive impairment since a right parietal stroke years ago, walks with a quad cane due to the stroke and osteoarthritis, and takes a diuretic and an angiotensin converting enzyme (ACE) inhibitor for congestive heart failure, which remains controlled. She lives alone in an apartment and is incontinent of urine, which she hates. She also complains of dizziness and tremor which, she says, impair her mobility more than the arthritis or stroke.

Which of the following strategies appeals to you as a potentially successful first step?

1. Contrive to let her know that dizziness and incontinence may be worsened by alcohol, among other things, after waiting a while to deflect suspicion from the nurse (turn to 8.5, page 133).

2. Call the local Alcoholics Anonymous chapter, and send a counsellor over to discuss the drinking problem with her (turn to 8.6, page 134).

3. Confront her at your next visit with her drinking problem, and recommend abstinence. Be firm in insisting that the drinking will harm her sooner, rather than later, and that she can get free of it using willpower (turn to 8.7, page 134).

4. Order blood alcohol, gamma GT, amylase, and stool occult blood to rule out complications of alcohol abuse (turn to 8.8, page 134).

Case 3

Henry Wheeler, aged 90, is an eccentric and remarkable man with prostate cancer and severe but burnt-out rheumatoid arthritis. He is a sort of ecclesiastical traveling salesman, who drives the minor highways of your region in a huge, perfectly maintained antique Chrysler, selling tracts, Bibles, and equipment to churches. He presents a government motor vehicle form, requesting a medical examination and your opinion as to his fitness to drive.

He has never had an accident and insists his driving is excellent. He never drives at night. His health has been good except as noted above, he takes no medication, and he never touches alcohol. Functional inquiry is negative.

Physical examination is normal, except for a Folstein Mini-Mental Status Examination score of 26 (he misses the date and two of the recalled objects and cannot write a sentence), his stony hard prostate and absent testicles from orchidectomy, and quite severe ulnar drift of the fingers of both hands, without any evidence of inflammation.

His eyesight is good, blood work and cardiogram are normal, and he walks without difficulty.

Should he be on the road? How do you handle this?

1. At age 90, nobody should be driving. The risk is simply too great. Lift his license (turn to 8.9, page 134).
2. This man is showing signs of cognitive impairment, and this impairs his ability to make decisions in traffic. License suspended (turn to 8.10, page 135).

3. He may be elderly, but there are no contraindications to driving here. See him again in one year (turn to 8.11, page 135).
4. Some of these features are worrisome, but none is absolutely inconsistent with safe driving. Recommend a road test; OK for another year if he appears to drive safely (turn to 8.12, page 135).

CHAPTER 9

Constipation, Fecal Incontinence, and Pressure Sores

Extended care (the skilled nursing facility) is considered by some physicians and other health care providers the least desirable type of geriatric work. Most removed from the traditional medical activities of diagnosis and cure, this world of very disabled people bores and otherwise repels physicians of a "quick fix, what's next" turn of mind. We enjoy extended care, however, because there is teamwork, often lots of room for improvement, and patients who really need our technical and humane excellence.

A lot of time in extended care is spent on three consequences of immobility: constipation, fecal incontinence, and pressure sores. A systematic and effective approach is as welcome and desirable here as in any area of health care. Some improved knowledge in these areas has done a lot to make care of these problems easier and better.

Our experience suggests that it is futile to argue over specific details of methodology in dealing with these problems. Once recognizing that a rational approach applied consistently usually will work well, we can quit worrying whether our methods are trendy and focus on a job done properly and consistently.

Constipation

We include constipation in this extended care–oriented chapter because its care is similar to that of fecal incontinence. All elderly people may get constipated, of course, but most relatively independent ones handle it without help. The current generation of elderly still fear infrequent bowel movements, as do some caregivers, for different reasons. Because we know that normal movement frequency is a very relative concept and we recognize true mechanical bowel obstruction in extended care patients as a rare, often preterminal event rather than a signal for aggressive action, we can reassure our colleagues and patients that everything will be just fine and explain that our rational approach will eventually bring results, no matter what the underlying problem.

The recipe presented here has worked a thousand times. If you have your own and are happy with it, skip this section and read on. If you need help, here's how it's done.

Eliminate Specific Constipation Causes

Two classes of drugs defeat normal bowel function: diuretics, which contribute to dehydration, and anticholinergic drugs, including tricyclic antidepressants, antihistamines, and narcotics. Both types of medication should be evaluated for their contribution on the positive side and perhaps eliminated as a trial to evaluate the need for them. Anything painful in the extreme lower digestive tract can stop bowel movements cold. Thrombosed hemorrhoids, fissures, skin problems, and strictures may prevent old people from voluntarily moving their bowels, with a presentation of chronic constipation as a result. Bowel obstruction is so much less common than constipation that it need be considered only briefly, especially if the patient is one whose treatment of mechanical obstruction would be palliative. Extreme constipation, called *pseudo-obstruction*, can present the same way, so a diagnostic work-up, usually not beyond serial plain films, may be necessary.

Assure Participation of Mother Nature

Nobody sentient can have escaped grasping the importance of fiber and bulk in the diet as promoters of normal bowel movements. There are still some elderly who carry a diagnosis of "colitis" from past decades and who are afflicted with the old low-fiber regime for functional bowel disease. Root vegetables are an important component of a high-fiber diet. Bran, prunes, not-overcooked vegetables, and grains are the other usual recommendations, familiar to everyone.

The epidemiology of fecal impaction is seasonal in our unit because of dehydration in the summer. Everyone, especially those on diuretics, needs to be presented with enough fluid to maintain stool consistency every day, but more than usual when the air temperature is high.

When the patient is immobile, the bowels are immobile. If moving around in bed is all someone can accomplish, it needs to be encouraged, as much as frequently sitting up in a chair, "paddling" around in a wheelchair, struggling daily to overcome standing and step-taking impairments, all assisted if the outdoors or other parts of an institutional environment are available for safe wandering. Abandoning efforts to maintain mobility brings a variety of trouble other than constipation down on the heads of caregivers and patients alike.

Clean Out and Regularize

Once drug rationalization and natural bowel-movers are assured, our approach features clearing out old fecal impaction and then taking whatever measures are required so that bowel movements occur when caregivers and patients want them to, not otherwise.

Enemas, suppositories, or laxatives are used in sufficient quantity to eliminate fecal impaction that is palpable rectally or abdominally or visible on a plain film. A laxative (ranging from magnesium hydroxide to magnesium hydroxide/mineral oil to lactulose or senna) is given at bedtime every 2 to 4 days. On the morning after, a suppository (glycerine or bisacodyl) is inserted immediately after breakfast, and the patient toileted or disimpacted at that time. If the result is more frequent or the stool more voluminous than desired, reduce the frequency, potency, or dose of the laxatives or suppositories. If it is less, increase. Trial and error will lead to a regime that works for each patient. Over many months, the potency of the preparations can be reduced, and possibly the evening laxative eliminated. Occasionally, a bowel will "train" with this regime, sufficient to permit intervention to stop altogether.

Be persistent. There's enough flexibility here to accommodate a wide range of normal.

Fecal Incontinence

Because caregiver morale is so critical to the well being of disabled patients, we seek and aggressively eliminate fecal incontinence continually. Nothing makes a family member at home or a professional in a facility dislike their task as much as dealing with "oozing" stool.

Extremely disabled people may have formed bowel movements in bed and simply be cleaned with a minimum of difficulty. We don't consider this fecal incontinence.

An easy mnemonic, FECAL, for reversible fecal incontinence causes can help:

Fecal impaction, the most common cause of incontinence in facilities.

Excess laxative, the most common cause in acute care.

Cognitive and behavioral problems. Very demented patients or those with an aggressive or vindictive side to their nature may use incontinence on caregivers as a means of negative expression.

All diarrhea causes, any of which can result in fecal incontinence.

Local anorectal problems, including adenomas, carcinomas, and neurological causes of sphincter tone loss.

The clinical circumstances will indicate whether fecal impaction or laxatives are likely to blame; and the "clean out and regularize" regimen suggested earlier will often work in impaction. Sigmoidoscopy may be necessary to assist in ruling out diarrhea causes or eliminate local tumors, which may be treatable.

Eventually, persistent loose bowel movement for which there is no identifiable or treatable cause can be controlled with loperamide or codeine, barring contraindications.

Pressure Sores

Although a marker for poor care if seen frequently, pressure sores can happen in excellent units as well. They are the result of skin injury, usually ischemic, contributed to by various causes. Anything preventing oxygen and nutrition from reaching the local tissue area (anemia, hypoxia, malnutrition, circulation compromised by atherosclerosis or diabetes) predisposes to skin damage. Edema, local infection, and the presence of moisture as urine or perspiration macerate and compromise the local tissue, further preparing for trouble.

Pressure of skeletal and visceral structures on compromised skin over a period of time, combined with the sideways tearing that occurs when the skeleton is moved while the skin stays stuck to the bed surface, results in the trauma or damage which creates a lesion.

These injuries begin with erythema and warmth for longer than 24 hours (Shea Grade I), continue with skin breakdown that penetrates to subcutaneous fat (Grade II), can continue into undermining between the fat and muscle, especially with excess shearing force (Grade III), and can end up with necrosis right to muscle or bone (Grade IV).

Prevention and treatment can be instituted using the mnemonic POINTS:

Pressure and shearing forces which can be relieved by frequent turning, special beds (including some new ones, which though expensive, can eliminate pressure sores dramatically), cushions, and care with lifting and moving to minimize the presence of lateral shearing.

Operate to debride necrotic tissue, using a simple scalpel, scissors, and forceps set. The presence of blood is not alarming and indicates viable tissue.

Infection must be treated if it is truly contributing to the problem. Clinical evidence of cellulitis indicates good topical or oral antibiotic treatment for gram positives (strep and staph), fecal gram negatives, and (if the wound is at all deep) anaerobes may be helpful. Mupirocin or polymyxin B/bacitracin can be used topically, metronidazole topically or orally, and cephalexin, erythromycin, or cotrimoxisole orally. Culturing pressure sores may be helpful in hospital situations where treatment has failed, otherwise it isn't often useful, since the organisms grown rarely correspond to the pathogens.

Nursing care includes the extremely wide range of old and new methods and products that have been used as dressings and claimed as miracle cures for pressure sores over a long period of time. New polymer and colloid products do seem, in well-conducted studies, to be more effective than most other methods. Strong chemicals damage tissue and shouldn't be used. Beyond this, any carefully applied benign dressing will be effective eventually at promoting healing.

Treat the general condition. If conditions such as anemia, malnutrition, or congestive heart failure are remediable, their care may speed healing.

Surgery may be necessary if all else fails, including flaps and grafts, which are usually done by a specialist.

Clinical Exercise

Case 1

Beryl Bachop lives at home in an apartment. She is 81 years of age, a widow, and suffers from osteoarthritis and congestive heart failure. She complains to you of being unable to have regular bowel movements and asks what she might use as treatment.

She says she eats a healthy diet, takes her medications (furosemide 40 mg po once daily, acetaminophen 325 mg with codeine 8 mg 1–2 po q4h prn pain, enalapril 5 mg po od) regularly, and is as active as her condition will permit, including daily walks. She still drives a car. She has no other digestive symptoms, no shortness of breath, and finds that her pain pills are adequate for the arthritis.

The physical examination is negative. Jugular venous pressure is below the sternal angle. Respiratory rate is 16, and blood pressure is 110/70 sitting.

How would you start in formulating a strategy to help this patient?

1. Find out what she means by "healthy" diet. Many old people subsist on tea and toast, believing they are well nourished (turn to 9.1, page 135).
2. Stools for occult blood, colon contrast evaluation, and possible GI referral are necessary to rule out serious digestive pathology (turn to 9.2, page 136).

3. Start a well-organized regimen of evening laxative and morning suppository, carefully monitoring progress to assure normal regular bowel movements (turn to 9.3, page 136).
4. Try to reduce furosemide and codeine, hoping they are contributing to the problem (turn to 9.4, page 136).

Case 2

Heinrich Krupp is a 86-year-old stroke victim living in an extended care unit. During a routine multidisciplinary conference, facility care aides bemoan his oozing fecal incontinence. He is not on a laxative regime, the stool is soft and extremely foul, he eats well and does not appear to be in pain, and there is no history of previous bowel disease.

He is not on any medication, and was discharged from acute care following a 6-week admission to the plastic surgery service, where a flap procedure to heal a stubborn pressure wound was complicated by recurrent infection, eventually eradicated by infectious disease specialists.

There are no physical findings in the abdomen, and digital rectal examination is really unremarkable, except for soft dark brown stool.

Assuming there is high fecal impaction, you arrange a laxative/suppository bowel clean out over 3 days, and return to find the problem worse still. What next?

1. Organize sigmoidoscopic examination, with suction to look for local anal–rectal causes and rule out inflammatory bowel disease (turn to 9.5, page 136).
2. Start loperamide 2 mg po qid (turn to 9.6, page 137).
3. Send stool for *C. difficile* toxin and/or start metronidazole 500 mg po bid (turn to 9.7, page 137).
4. Begin regularizing measures with evening laxatives and morning suppository every 3 days (turn to 9.8, page 137).

Case 3

Nursing in your extended care unit requests some help in healing a chronic ulcer over the sacrum of a thin, elderly woman under your care. She has severe dementia and Parkinson's disease, and has not left her bed for many months since stiffness and seating problems made it impossible for her to be up, even during the day.

Looking at the ulcer, it is 2 cm in diameter, and the skin moves freely over underlying exposed muscle. Current treatment has involved twice daily soaks with 1/4 strength Dakins' solution and turning the patient in bed every few hours.

The wound is apparently painless, there is no odor, and it looks clean. Surrounding tissue appears healthy, but there is an irregular rim of dark tissue around the edge measuring several millimeters.

Choose your first, second, and third strategies from the options presented below:

1. Start turning her more frequently (turn to 9.9, page 137).
2. Acquire a scalpel, scissors, and forceps, and debride the edges of the wound (turn to 9.10, page 137).
3. Move up the concentration of Dakins' to full strength and increase the frequency of soaks (turn 9.11, page 138).
4. Culture the wound, particularly the undermined section, and send for C&S including anaerobes (turn to 9.12, page 138).
5. Lose the Dakins' and switch to saline dressings (turn to 9.13, page 138).
6. Check her hemoglobin, institute multiple vitamins, and try to improve her nutrition (turn to 9.14, page 138).

CHAPTER 10

Difficult Behavior

Care of elderly people, whether provided by professionals or family, is always made more challenging by persisting difficult-to-handle behavior. Dealing with this clinical situation is such a huge priority in practical geriatrics that most professionals must at some point learn to evaluate and treat it.

What is it? Difficult behavior is apparently a final common pathway of various neurological and psychological problems common in mentally disabled people. We are nearly always talking about the cognitively impaired here, and usually those moderately or severely cognitively impaired. Descriptive definitions of the problem use words such as *agitation*, *sundowning*, *aggressiveness*, and *wandering*. Behavior is then further categorized by primary caregivers as shouting, escaping, fighting with care, hitting out, rummaging, throwing food, banging, howling, biting, breaking things, and so on.

Naming the exact behavior may not always lead to useful diagnosis and treatment, but the problem is often presented by a frustrated and unhappy caregiver in some specific terms. For health professionals and for the patient, the potential cost of allowing difficult behavior to continue is loss of stable caregiving, possible abuse, institutionalization, escalation of expense, and some real suffering. We need to deal with agitation, and deal with it quickly.

Approaches to Diagnosis

Like most presentations in geriatrics, difficult behavior may be caused or worsened by one or more remediable factors. There are several systems for quickly reviewing these.

First, possible contributors can be classified as biological, psychological, social, and environmental to help organize a search for them. Illness, medication, and pain would be examples of biological realities that increase frustration and anger in a demented person, and which might be treatable. Any psychological illness (schizophrenia, mania, depression, personality disorder) can start or worsen agitation, as can any psychological symptom overlying a state of cognitive impairment (anxiety, depression, panic).

Socially, the people around the patient (caregiver, other residents, professionals, occasionally others), may be doing things counterproductive to behavior control, inadvertently or not. We get at these situations by tactful, nonjudging, willing-to-help questioning of everyone involved. Changing behavior or changing people may help and may be difficult. Circumstances in the patient's past may condition a reaction to people or situations. An elderly retired prospector, for example, fights with care because he has not been undressed by a female since age 2. Environment changes, such as a move to a facility, an ostensibly socializing but (to a sensitive resident) chaotic and frightening program situation, darkness, bright lights, silence, loud noise, too big a space, or too small a space are all possible creators of fear and bewilderment and contributors to agitation. Modifying these can be difficult, too, and the process is one of trial and error.

Working with a medical-type model, one can also fairly quickly evaluate behaviorally difficult people for the presence of common contributing diagnoses. The mnemonic "D is for agitation" can help. *Dolor* is Latin for pain, which can have any cause, may be completely occult in someone who can't communicate, and is very important because it is treatable. Look carefully for injuries, medical musculoskeletal pain causes, and abdominal pain. The circumstances of the agitation may help: fighting and shouting when diapers are applied may indicate hip osteoarthritis, refusing to transfer can be knee pain, noisy bedtime might mean gastroesophageal reflux disease present. Trials of therapy can be rewarding.

Any medication (*drug*) can cause agitation. Frequent offenders are selective serotonin reuptake inhibitors (especially fluoxetine), any neuroleptic that gives rise to akathisia, and any anticholinergic drug that contributes to delirium. Try stopping them.

Delirium can be a very hard find in advanced dementia. The setting of illness is the most consistent clue, a change in behavior without obvious causes raises suspicion, and the sixth sense of a caregiver or health professional who knows the patient may be the only indications. Look carefully and quickly for common causes (see Chapter 6).

DSM reminds us that people with history of major psychiatric disease who have been in institutions, on psychiatric medications, or had electroconvulsive therapy (ECT) throughout their lives, may benefit from treatment directed at the old diagnosis after they become demented. Others develop treatable psychological conditions with their disease, organically or secondarily. Loxapine may work for behavior control, but specific treatment may work if a psychological illness can be identified.

Drainage helps recall fecal impaction and urinary retention, which are common, easy to rule out, and supertreatable. Don't miss them.

Disputes or stressful circumstances between the agitated person and other residents or caregivers can be a cause of difficult behavior. It is necessary to spend the time finding out how it feels to look after this person and to be cared for by this caregiver. Dementia caregiving can seem pretty thankless, and demented people can have troubling ideas about race, gender, intention, or appropriateness of those who look after them. Approach these situations with a very open mind; an abusive caregiver is still a caregiver, and a little understanding and encouragement go a long way.

Dementia's biological changes can produce personality and behavior difficulty independent of coexisting other causes. The frontal lobe is affected, leading to disinhibition, and the biological seat of personality can be affected by the disease process.

In practice, aggression may be in response to recurring difficulties, and therefore primarily social or environmental, or spontaneous, and therefore likely biological or psychological.

Approach to Managing Difficult Behavior

We often find people who care for these patients, quite understandably, at their wits' end. They may already have taken steps to terminate or modify their responsibility or be thinking about doing so. We need to attempt to suspend the collapse of caregiving by taking immediate effective action. Provide plenty of reassurance and explanation, and promise (and deliver) a prompt reevaluation. Use an effective dose of medication right away. Explain the titration process. Negotiate a respite. Arrange for a strictly limited hospital admission of a few days. Whatever it takes, show responsible partnership and then get on with the diagnostic and therapeutic job.

Using the aforementioned lists, after a history, physical, and lab evaluation are underway, make your best guess as to the agitation cause and start tentative treatment. A temperature and crackles in the right base are pneumonia; treatment is antibiotics and loxapine. A boardlike silent abdomen in a terminal patient is treated with parenteral morphine and possibly loxapine. A trial of antidepressants in someone with a history of the disease may also require benzodiazepines or loxapine while you wait for a response to therapy.

If there is a central message in the primary care of frail elderly people, it is that frequent reevaluation is the essence of the process. Get back to the facility, the bedside, or the home within a day or a few days, see what is going on, and modify the approach appropriately. Diagnosis is so tentative and outcomes so varied that this is technically necessary, as well as important for reassurance and information-gathering.

Monitoring in a facility can be difficult. Professional caregivers must understand the treatment plan, the expected outcome, and their responsibility for reporting. Arrange monitoring using a form in the chart if possible but allow for written description, and seek person-to-person spoken reports if you can get them.

Treatment by behavior sometimes works. If nurses are using a program, get involved and help. If not, try to create one ad hoc. Unfortunately, demented people, unable to learn, must have their behavior modified newly each time. Avoid unrealistic expectations.

Drug treatment is nearly always helpful and very seldom harmful on balance, given always that the prescriber is responsible and constantly vigilant about evaluating adverse consequences and benefit. One might read that last sentence a second time.

With medication, we choose our side effects. Benzodiazepines produce sedation, contribute to falling, and impair remaining mental sharpness, but they buy time by controlling anger and fear to allow a thorough evaluation. Short-acting drugs with few metabolites are best. Temazepam, alprazolam, and oxazepam are the ones we use at present; others are also appropriate. Flurazepam, diazepam, chlordiazepoxide, and lorazepam are long half-life drugs with complex metabolites, probably unsafe at any dose in the elderly. Using benzodiazepines "prn" has not worked for us; an approach borrowed from pain control is better, where a basic regular dose is given, and a prn "breakthrough" permitted.

Longer-term behavior control and sometimes first line success can often be achieved using neuroleptics. These dopamine antagonists seem to diminish terrifying bewilderment that may exist both in major psychotic states and cognitive impairment. Each drug bristles with potential problems, mandating an even more careful than usual follow-up and titration. Haloperidol is very effective, but it can also freeze patients into disabling Parkinsonism and create bewildering akathisia. Thioridazine has fewer movement disorder problems, but it is antihistaminic (drowsiness producing), anticholinergic (confusogenic), and antiadrenergic (productive of orthostatic hypotension). Risperidone is a complex drug with few direct side effects but many drug interactions and late problems. At the moment, our experience is limited, and specialists use this drug for us.

Still a best compromise is loxapine, with mild antihistaminic effects, mild to moderate antidopaminergic side effects, and fairly good antipsychotic potency. Long-term use may lead to late movement disorders and necessitate a decrease.

The news in behavior control with drugs is antiepileptics. Phenytoin and carbamazepine have been used in the past. After some initial success with carbamazepine and some catastrophes with phenytoin, we now use valproate, starting in low doses of 125 mg po once daily, and titrate very slowly to behavior change. Liver enzyme problems and digestive symptoms can occur. This drug can be very helpful in patients who don't respond to loxapine or can't tolerate it or where a mood disorder is suspected as part of the diagnostic cluster.

Used in psychiatry before neuroleptics were invented, morphine has occasionally been very effective when nothing else works. These may be occult pain patients; in any case, addiction and tolerance would be tiny prices to pay if comfort and continued caregiving could be purchased in no other way. There is literature to support beta blockers in this setting. Our experience is limited, but these drugs would be a reasonable choice in hypertension and angina patients with behavior problems.

Clinical Exercise

Leopold Evier is a 76-year-old disabled chef living in a veteran's extended care facility. Feistily demented at the best of times, the facility staff report Leopold recently to be unmanageable. Before, he made obscene remarks during nursing care. Now, he desperately fights routine attempts to clean him and put him in the wheelchair. Before, he disrupted peace and quiet in the public area and was frequently confined to his ward room; now, in spite of having been placed in a private room, he throws objects and stool at visitors and caregivers and has caused expensive damage to room equipment and furniture. There is no past psychiatric history.

He has vascular dementia, scoring 10 out of 30 on the Folstein Mini-Mental Status Examination 6 months ago. Strokes have lead to hemiplegia and severe balance problems, so he is chair-fast. Two months ago, he was in acute hospital for a short time because of new onset of congestive heart failure; this is now controlled.

His medications are oxazepam 15 mg po at hs, furosemide 40 mg po od, cilazapril 7.5 mg po od, potassium 20 mEq 2 tabs po od, ranitidine 150 mg po bid, and acetaminophen with codeine as required for pain.

On functional inquiry, his bowels and urine are fine, and there is no evidence of obvious illness in any of his other systems.

The staff now state that they are pretty fed up with Leopold. If this trouble continues, they plan to transfer him to a nearby former government mental hospital, now a psychogeriatric unit.

Effective and intelligent first action on your part would be:

1. Conduct physical and laboratory evaluation, and (depending on the outcome) consider neuroleptic medication (turn to 10.1, page 138).

2. Loxapine 5.0 mg po bid now; physical and laboratory evaluation to follow (turn to 10.2, page 139).

3. Interview caregivers to determine what triggers the aggressive behavior, whether certain behaviors and approaches are less stimulating to him, and what his known previous interests were, in case evoking these will help (turn to 10.3, page 139).

4. CT head scan, psychiatry referral, and possibly neuropsychological testing to determine whether a new stroke or some other central nervous system (CNS) problem has precipitated the difficulty or if Mr. Evier is suffering depression or psychosis (turn to 10.4, page 139).

Treated with loxapine 5.0 po bid for a few days, Mr. Evier is less agitated but still fearful and distracted. His respiratory rate is 16, jugular venous pressure below the sternal angle, chest clear, blood pressure is 100/60 lying (unobtainable standing), heart rate 100 regular, abdomen soft, no palpable pain in trunk or extremities, and no change in focal neurological findings. Sodium is 126, potassium 4.3, creatinine 180, and his chest x-ray is clear.

He refuses to cooperate with mental status testing and makes internally consistent comments unrelated to questions or the circumstances of the examination.

What next?

1. Increase the loxapine, and monitor carefully (turn to 10.5, page 139).

2. Renal ultrasound to rule out obstructive azotemia cause (turn to 10.6, page 140).

3. Reduce furosemide to 20 mg po once daily and observe for congestive heart failure (CHF); if none after 4 days, discontinue furosemide, along with potassium, and observe behavior, respiratory rate, and electrolytes (turn to 10.7, page 140).

4. Change loxapine to 5 mg po tid prn agitation to determine the real need for medication (turn to 10.8, page 140).

Mr. Evier calmed down over a week, and his blood pressure and renal function returned with oral rehydration. Loxapine was tapered and discontinued, and he returned to his offensive but otherwise harmless antisocial baseline.

Geriatrics Topics and Questions

C. Special Topics

CHAPTER 11

The Team and Case Management

Everyone agrees that evaluation and care of geriatric patients is complex and sometimes difficult. They don't just have pneumonia, they become confused, can't walk or dress, lose continence, mix up their drugs, and don't eat *because* they have pneumonia. To expect one professional to provide all the care required isn't reasonable, hence the multidisciplinary team.

Teams have existed in geriatrics and other settings for decades. Recently, the process and dynamics of teams have been studied and evaluated systematically. Here we describe the team in general terms, discuss what it does, and address the role of the case manager, also known as the care coordinator.

A definition of a team is necessarily loose. Any time you systematically collaborate with another professional to pool your expertise, a team exists. This is also true in large and complex teams that manage dozens of clients simultaneously and employ numerous professionals full-time.

There is no substitute in any cooperative enterprise for mutual respect. Healthy teams' members know and understand one another's strengths and weaknesses (personally and professionally), overlook unimportant peculiarities and deficiencies, and frequently discuss the process and any problems in a neutral, forthright way.

An effective care process requires someone's keeping track of what's going on. If the same job is done twice, resources are wasted and conflict can take root; if a step is missed, the whole process may be weakened. Keeping track of things (case management) is very important; it entails responsibility (if things aren't organized, you haven't done your job) with ownership (you have a right to know about everything that is going on with this client). In primary care, case management looks to us like a 24-hour job.

Team Members

Geriatric multidisciplinary teams traditionally include a nurse, a doctor, and a social worker. This reflects the fact that direct health care, diagnosis, prescription and titration of medication, and the organization of community supports are usually unavoidable tasks. If this group (or at least the functions it performs) is at the center, a next-closest concentric circle of professional functions would include mobility evaluation and support (a physiotherapist); detailed evaluation and assistance with activities of daily living (an occupational therapist); monitoring, organizing, and providing medication and advice about its use to prescriber and recipient (a pharmacist); and detailed surveillance of nutrition (a nutritionist). Psychologists, financial assistants, orthotists, podiatrists, various medical specialists, and everyone else might form a third circle.

So much for the professionals. The informal team includes nonprofessional helpers, the family, and the patient themselves. Effectiveness often depends on communication between the professional group and its organization and activities and this informal team. Responsibility rests with the case manager. Picture the concentric circles with the patient and family at the very center, and things work even better.

Who should case manage? We have not found that any health professional is generically better suited than any other. This is, however, a special role and requires a special capability for balancing the gestalt of overall trends and directions with the sometimes quite numerous details of care. The best case managers are unfailingly bifocal: quite comfortable simultaneously with the big picture and the small print.

Team Roles

What one does in a team is partly defined by one's professional role. Physiotherapists diagnose musculoskeletal problems and improve mobility. Social workers evaluate community function and arrange support, and nurses monitor health status and intervene to maintain it. But everyone is a geriatric professional, and the doctor can perfectly well measure joint range of movement and assess cognitive function, the social worker understands the importance of medication compliance, and the psychologist may help in an interview to deal with the impact of cognitive impairment on a caregiver. Depending on your precise circumstances, a "zone defense" situation where professional roles are flexible and everyone moves over a little to help out may be a useful way of seeing the team's function.

The balance here is between a rigid group with professionals blindered into inflexible roles and a chaotic mess where team members overfunction their way into turf problems and redundancy. Never allow lack of an apparently essential professional, however, to stop you from developing and being a team and doing a comprehensive job.

Team Process

The care process may be consultative, as when a geriatric evaluation unit sees someone and eventually returns them to the community, or primary, as when a physician and nurse work with a mental health agency or adult day center to manage problems long term. The process is roughly concerned with comprehensive geriatric assessment (see Chapter 2) and management in either case.

The fullest possible comprehensive geriatric assessment (see Chapter 2) is mandatory, at least once, usually at intake. We believe it can have any professional focus but would eventually include evaluation by all relevant core professionals and be quite thorough. A meeting next occurs, at which everyone potentially involved discusses the case and plans the course of evaluation and care to be pursued. At this point, a case manager can be designated, to assume documentary and global directive responsibility. It is agreed which types of professional assessment other than that by core professionals is necessary, and this is arranged, including referrals outside the team. However named and recorded, a problem list is developed, and each item on it will give rise to plans for care.

Repeated conferences are the essence of effective team function. Crises are recognized and dealt with. The business of the conference is review of the problem list, reformulation of plans, scheduling of what everyone will do, and setting of short time-lines.

Patients leave the process by death or choice in primary care and when the evaluation is complete in a consultative team. Either way, the process is difficult, important, expensive, and potentially useful and so needs to be documented. Documentation needn't be time-consuming, but it must be usable, and it must be done.

Troubleshooting

It is not always Friday, the sun isn't always shining (where we live at least), and the home team occasionally goes down to defeat. A team manager (as distinct from case manager) may encounter problems and needs to be creative to keep things running smoothly.

Conflict in teams usually involves failure of the aforementioned process of role definition and role sharing. Most conflicts contain an element of overfunctioning on someone's part; leadership is a touchy issue for some people, and there is no substitute for repeated clear definition of what everyone is doing.

A team must define whom it cares for precisely enough to avoid wasting time. If you don't want alcohol abusers or unstable cardiac patients, say so. If your strength is in mental health, let the referral base know about it.

Geriatrics can seem frustrating at times. This sense of running in dry sand may get to team members and create a false sense of futility. Our three cures for unhappy team members are education, professional team development, and socializing. Members returning from professional conferences are rejuvenated and can enrich team knowledge. Formal or informal introspection to better understand and develop the team's activities can refocus everyone. When in doubt, if all else fails (or just to celebrate), throw a party.

Clinical Exercise

You have landed a new job: medical director of a multidisciplinary geriatric evaluation and management outreach team in your town. So far, only the team manager, (a nurse with extensive geriatric and community experience) and yourself have been hired. The team's overseeing agency envisions multidisciplinary evaluation of challenging frail elderly people referred by various sources, with primary care returning to the family physician and other community care givers once your job is done.

The budget is limited. Assuming the director is a full-time administrator, whom (in terms of professional roles) will you advise hiring? (Turn to 11.1, page 141.)

In organizing the team process, you are asked to recommend a method of case management. How would you handle this? (Turn to 11.2, page 141.)

Can you outline 5 or 6 steps in the team process, that you would consider essential to the success of this program? (Turn to 11.3, page 141.)

The team is up and functioning. There is a good but not overwhelming flow of referrals, and the process appears to run smoothly. The clinical nurse, however, confides to you on the way back from a home visit that she has a problem with the unit director. One of the clinical nurse's case-management patients was discharged from the program by the director because the client's family failed to bring her to the day unit three times in a row. The clinical nurse feels the director should stick to administration and leave clinical decisions alone. Any suggestions to help with this conflict? (Turn to 11.4, page 142.)

CHAPTER 12

Home Care and Caregiver Support

There may be some truth to the idea that a traditional health care system, centered in institutions and bent on precise diagnosis and cure, is spinning its expensive wheels in attempting to solve the problems of some complicated dependent old people. Often these patients neither want nor can benefit from hospital-style care. If the effort and time now sometimes wasted in trying to convince them to accept it anyway were spent improving their custodial care at home, might we all be further ahead?

Several types of care at home have evolved in response to this. Hospital stays for operations, myocardial infarcts, and intravenous medication are radically shortened with replacement by services at home. The elderly, either briefly in crisis or more lengthily requiring chronic disease support, fulfill their needs without abandoning the psychosocial and (to the system) economic benefits of staying home. Dying patients especially need and enjoy this service. The emergency room, long an inappropriate safety net for failed primary care, arranges short, intensive home support when appropriate, instead of a hospital admission, ill-informed acute medical care, and a belated, inept look at social and chronic care problems from within the hospital.

Home care looks positive from several points of view. The quality can be better than institutional care, if futility, danger, expense, and the morbidity of hospital-enforced immobility are considered, along with the privacy and dignity of staying at home. Are new studies that show patient preference, patient satisfaction, quicker recovery, and less morbidity with care at home valid and applicable to most patients? At least it now seems that home care is neither dangerous nor neglectful. We may be nearing a time when the home will replace the hospital as the default setting in final illness.

Since waking up to health care's unsustainable expense, we have discovered that caring for people at home can provide benefits beyond cost-savings. The reason home care makes sense is that money formerly inefficiently applied to the problems of dependent old people through traditional institutions can be much more effectively used by keeping close track of health problems at home, so that health deterioration is anticipated, prepared for, and dealt with in a way the patient prefers.

Home Care Doctors

General physicians interested in geriatrics are getting out of the hospital and office. This changed behavior is not for everybody. Caring for people in their homes doesn't work without a multidisciplinary team (see Chapter 11), and case management, which is beyond the time resources of most family physicians, must be done by someone. If the case manager takes true responsibility for health care, the doctor must be ready to let go of some of the executive-command authority traditionally associated with the job. It isn't reasonable to use a physician's valuable and focused time and skills for carrying the documentary and traffic-directing responsibility of a set of problems that are mainly nonmedical.

Doctors who want the professional satisfaction of being comprehensive, really using their hard-won diagnostic and therapeutic skills, and meticulously following up the many difficult problems of older patients at home may want to consider payment methods other than good old fee-for-service. Finally, the comfort and order of a well-appointed office may disappear, to be replaced by chaotic-appearing adult day centers, busy nursing homes, community health clinics, and a car.

Tools of the Home Care Trade

Certain venues, attitudes, and patterns of care lend themselves to looking after people at home and can be usefully assimilated into a home health care practice. The adult day center, traditionally a place of respite for caregivers and socialization for disabled older people, is often the best site for professional visits to monitor treatment outcome, and for special clinics as well. Anticipation is the essence of good primary home care. If you aren't on top of what's happening with the client, unproductive visits to the emergency room will persist, and improved privacy, dignity, and other home benefits may not materialize.

Nobody expects to predict everything. Falls, strokes, undiagnosed breathlessness, and sudden aggressive behavior are daily facts of life in a home care setting. The difference is that an effective home care service responds immediately, on a 24-hour basis, to the home. In a setting of carefully worked-out advance directives and a mutually accepted understanding of priorities for care (whether for comfort only, admission to hospital under specified circumstances, or immediate comfort with community investigation when convenient), a crisis can often be tentatively named, a plan for evaluation and treatment established, symptoms controlled, and everyone reassured on the spot.

None of this is possible unless the person responding to a crisis call is informed and capable. A single medical record, which is the responsibility of the case manager, must exist and travel, preferably electronically. The patients are difficult and their problems numerous. Home care is no place for professionals to hide if they are not confident of their clinical skills.

Indications for use of scarce health resources can be rationalized in a good home care program. Planned or crisis respite, short convalescence, and certain investigations might be a particular person's predesignated reasons for admission to hospital or nursing home. A nurse, in touch with a doctor by frequent conferences, can be as effective as the physician at determining the consequences of a Parkinson's disease prescription or of a corticosteroid injection. Understanding this through repeated experience can reassure many older people who might otherwise require the placebo magic of the black bag and white coat. Doctors doing home care are true generalists, comfortable with common psychiatric and internal medicine problems and the comprehensive handling of complex medication used to treat them. Medical specialists should never be consulted to save time or buy a clinical update at patient or system expense but only to answer a specific critical question or to help solve a truly difficult problem.

Difficult older people whose real, organic, and multiple problems are fairly straightforward but who also suffer psychosocial problems may be passed back and forth among well-intentioned specialists who recognize that they have little to offer when caught within a hospital setting. One of the benefits of home care by a general physician is that these perfectly legitimate deficiencies of specialized doctors are not a problem.

As in team dynamics (see Chapter 11), the conference is the center of the home care service. Everyone needs to know the status of each patient in his or her care, and an hour around a table with coffee Monday morning prepares primary providers for the week and informs them about the on-call events of the weekend. Regular conferences control the pace of all aspects of care.

Medication, its changes, the evaluation of its good and bad effects, and constant negotiation with its recipient is an absolutely unavoidable part of care of dependent old people. Everyone working in geriatrics knows that a poorly-complied-with drug regimen is worse than none at all. Whatever it takes to communicate, assure, and monitor correct medication-taking is a necessary first step to effective therapeutics at home.

Enter, therefore, the caregiver. Dealt with shortly in greater detail, the person who lives with and looks after a dependent older person is at least as important a focus as that person themselves.

Certain clients (like certain health professionals) just aren't right for home care. Those feeling themselves inalienably entitled to ambulance, a beeping monitored heartbeat, and daily parade of teaching specialists at the end of their lives will not be happy with the homely comforts of a nurse, social worker, or simple general practitioner at the home bedside, no matter how comprehensively these professionals may provide for their biological and psychological needs. This must be evaluated at the outset, and everyone must be absolutely in agreement. Every elderly person cared for at home must discuss, understand, and decide on issues such as cardiopulmonary resuscitation, the importance of comfort versus prolonging life, and the delegation of a substituted decision-maker. Great care must be observed if you are dealing with someone incompetent, properly to evaluate and decide on these issues. Err on the side of caution and tradition. Families and others may belatedly raise doubts about what was and wasn't done after someone dies comfortably in his own bed.

The Caregiver: Helping the Helpers

Literature supports the idea that outcomes in the frail elderly depend on caregiver characteristics. Therefore, effective home care services focus heavily on supporting these important individuals.

Caregivers must understand what they are up against. Groups of people in similar circumstances can quickly pass informal information and provide support. Information pamphlets and books are now available in enough variety to correspond to any level of interest and literacy. A home care team must designate someone to make sure knowledge gaps are closed, one-on-one, in the caregiver's home. The caregiver also requires understanding of the services being offered. Advance directives must carefully and repeatedly be discussed so that crisis misunderstanding is minimized.

Caregiving is unimaginably difficult at times. Group and individual sessions can help deal with frustration, grief, substance abuse issues, and the sense of isolation that arise routinely.

One of the most powerful strategies for maintaining caregiver effectiveness is respite. Recognize the relentless nature of the task, promise and deliver daily hours using home support or adult day center, and then use a facility or 24-hour in-home assistance to give a good, long holiday a couple of times a year.

Most caregivers are women. They may be employed at two jobs. Caregiving, though through biology and social tradition a female role, is as yet unpaid. Listen to needs, and use your knowledge and energy to cut through bureaucracy to get support to these essential people.

In a sense, the confidence and satisfaction of the caregiver is as accurate a report card as any on the effectiveness of your home care. If you deliver on your promises, admit your mistakes, come when you're called, and give the respect due to caregivers, they will contribute hugely to the success of your professional task.

Clinical Exercise

As a traditional office-based family physician, you are asked by a patient and his family about the advisability of his going into a nursing home. Arthritis and a stroke have made it difficult for him to do essential activities outside the home, and he now requires assistance with taking a bath and preparing his meals.

There exists a new agency in your town, which would, as an alternative to facility placement, assist this man to remain at home by providing in-home supports for personal care and by giving him further health maintenance and other services at an adult day center. The family wonders what you think of home care in general, assuming that the cost of the two options is not an issue. How might your patient benefit by staying at home? (Turn to 12.1, page 142.)

This patient decides to stay at home and try the home care agency. The agency sends you literature on its program, which includes primary medical care if it is required by the client. The gentleman and his family are pleased with your care and ask you to continue, in cooperation with the home care service. Unaccustomed to making house calls, what problems and potential changes in your practice style might you anticipate? (Turn to 12.2, page 142.)

CHAPTER 13

Nursing Home Care

Nursing home is a term used in geriatric literature to characterize a variety of different types of residences for older people. In the United Kingdom, Canada, and the United States, various names are used for various types of long-term care facilities. Generally, *senior citizen's housing*, or *personal care*, is a light-level facility where people live in apartments with or without provision of meals and supervision. *Nursing homes, ambulatory care facilities,* and *intermediate care facilities* refer to homes for frail elderly people needing daily assistance with activities of daily living, but who do not require 24-hour nursing care and who are usually ambulatory. *Extended care* or *skilled nursing facilities* are units in which elderly people are not independently ambulatory and require heavy personal support for activities of daily living (ADL) up to and including feeding.

Nursing homes are peculiar places, in that they combine characteristics of a home with those of a hospital. It is as incorrect and naive to imagine that an acute level of hospital care is available here as it is to believe that the health problems of the residents will not interfere with a homey atmosphere.

In many places, there is a trend toward disabled older people remaining in their homes. This means that the acuity, disability, age, and cognitive impairment of nursing home residents is, on average, on the rise. A very physically disabled person who is cognitively intact can spend the night at home alone, as long as help can be summoned. Severely cognitively impaired people who are physically capable, however, do need 24-hour supervision. Facilities look more and more like homes for demented people.

Very demented people who remain sufficiently physically capable to wander or those whose psychological problems create disturbance and danger are best managed in "special care" units. Staff members trained in dementia behavior management and a physical plant that combines safety and a secure perimeter will avoid some of the worst problems that can occur when difficult demented people and the merely physically frail cohabit.

Entering a nursing home can be a terribly sensitive time in someone's life. The term *relocation stress* encompasses all the negative responses to this critical situation. Caregivers need to be especially attentive to and supportive of old people who are having problems in the early weeks of a nursing home stay. Like children, cognitively impaired elderly people see through patronizing superficial reassurances that the facility is a wonderful, cheery, warm, and friendly place.

Nursing Home Characteristics

The people who live in nursing homes probably need a more "geriatric" style of care than any other single group. They are the frailest and most aged of patients, suffer from the greatest variety of multiple pathology, and take the most medication. Our goals for care are here most radically shifted away from a traditional disease-eradication model used in a younger adult population.

The goal of facility care is to maximize and to maintain independent function and comfort. Multiply pathological people sometimes suffer more from unrealistic efforts at cure than from health problems themselves. There is a fine line, however, between diagnostic and therapeutic nihilism and sloppiness and a careful, case-by-case evaluation of the potential impact of medical care on symptoms and independence. When a care professional decides that nothing further should be done, ask why. If the answer emphasizes age or sounds vague, take a closer look.

Disabled people depend on caregivers, and their families are often part of the health decision-making process. The right to self-determination is truly at risk in this situation.

Routines and expediency can easily replace the respect we owe to and intend for older patients. Someone whose dementia prevents them from understanding the issues in a cardiac arrest resuscitation decision may still understand enough to delegate a substituted decision-maker. Decision-making incapacity is often partial.

Decisions must be made in advance. Most facilities have a policy requiring that residents request various degrees of intervention in the event of a change in their health status. Typically, four degrees are offered: full hospital care up to and including intensive care and life support, hospital admission short of intensive care, treatment for cure in the facility, and treatment for comfort. The question of cardiac arrest resuscitation may be addressed separately or understood to be part of the highest degree of intervention only. Resuscitation is never appropriate in an unwitnessed cardiac arrest. Clinical situations may fall through the cracks between these degrees of intervention. Hip fracture repair and cataract surgery may be appropriate for a "cure in facility" resident, and an overwhelming neurological catastrophe may render a planned rush to the intensive care unit (ICU) inappropriate. Still, the degrees of intervention guidelines serve as indications of the resident's wishes. When in doubt, the previous knowledgeable delegation by the resident of a substituted decision-maker is extremely helpful.

Physicians routinely balance the information to be gained from investigations and the benefit of invasive treatment against the inconvenience, time, and discomfort associated with ambulance and taxi trips, waiting room ennui, and shuffling around hospitals and laboratories. In facilities, we lean toward keeping residents at home and using our clinical judgment. It is part of the challenge of nursing home care that these decisions must be made time and time again, individually, case-by-case.

The Doctor in the Nursing Home

Physicians working in a community with only one or two facilities are fortunate. They avoid the dilemma faced by their urban colleagues, whose community patients may be admitted to any of widely scattered facilities and continue to require visits and care. The "house doctor" model of care, in which a physician accumulates a number of patients in a facility and takes over the care of many patients from other physicians, may make better and more consistent care feasible. The other medical model (where patients are scattered all over town) preserves continuity of care but perhaps at too great a cost in loss of consistency.

Facilities often appoint or employ a medical director or coordinator. This physician is responsible for the quality of all medical care and normally oversees the compliance with standards of care by his colleagues. In the United States, the medical director may play a role in assisting with the commercial success of the facility by providing or encouraging admissions. Certain conflicts may arise. Ideally, the medical director is responsible for quality of care first and either cares for no residents in the facility or does a sufficiently exemplary job that the issue of evaluating his or her own care quality does not arise.

Physicians and other professionals are increasingly exposed to nursing homes in their training programs. A teaching nursing home may enjoy improved staff morale, better professional standards, and a somewhat shinier self-image. A great opportunity for teaching and learning collaborative care exists. Unlearning of some of the harmful chauvinism that is still occasionally seen in professional schools is a further benefit to everyone.

Whatever role the doctor plays, certain types of medical nursing home visits occur repeatedly. The initial patient evaluation, which may take several weeks, involves putting together the database and gathering old records. Former physicians who do not plan to continue a new resident's care needn't pretend to do a physical examination. Instead, they can provide valuable background information to the new doctor, who can then evaluate the patient.

When a new problem arises, a physician must be available within an hour or so and make a decision about urgency and need for a visit. Thorough documentation assists physicians on call who may not know the patient. Since every intervention creates a potential adverse outcome, the follow-up visit may be the most important of all. It needs to be scheduled following every drug prescription or dose change.

Finally, "stable" nursing home patients require routine surveillance, perhaps monthly to every six months (depending on complexity and frailty) and some sort of periodic evaluation should be done perhaps once or twice a year. This can be done by the attending physician or by the medical director. It should include updating evaluation of cognition, ADL performance, medication appropriateness, advance directives, and the medical problem list. There is no consensus on whether a traditional head-to-toe physical examination and routine laboratory evaluation of nursing home patients is of value. Influenza and pneumococcus immunization and tuberculosis status update are valuable.

Documentation

A nursing home record that is illegible, locked in the doctor's office, low quality, or out of date is worse than useless. These very complicated patients require an excellent record for even adequate care.

The record can only be useful if it contains certain elements. A problem list, ideally accessible to all disciplines, should exist somewhere and be well marked and up to date. Each discipline makes succinct progress notes. They may be multidisciplinary and mixed or separated by discipline, but they must be legible and understandable to everyone. A list of medications is important, but a clear notation of the justification for each drug is more valuable still. Cognition and ADL as basic parameters of resident function should be available somewhere on the chart, and the advance directives, including substituted decision-maker, need to be easily accessible to people dealing with an emergency. Records of consultations, hospital discharges, and laboratory evaluations complete the picture. Because care occurs in the facility, the document needs to be there. Physicians who guard their nursing home patients' records in an office file are probably not visiting or are just "popping by." The facility must be prepared to fax or copy and send out information with patients who are transferred, admitted to the hospital, or referred to specialists.

The old but rapidly changing relationship between doctors and nurses, complete with all its problems, is nowhere in sharper focus than in the facility. The scene is unlike a hospital, where physicians traditionally claim team leadership. The nursing home may be seen as a nurses' shop, which may be what makes some doctors so uncomfortable there. The patience and professionalism of the best of us is tested in numerous situations because, unlike the hospital, the nursing home has no tradition of convenient collaborative interdisciplinary routines.

Physicians are usually available in the early morning and just before supper, whereas nurses tend to have time in the late afternoon shift, or mid-evening. This gives rise to all sorts of problems, including the doctor's visit at mealtime (when nurses are least available) and the nursing telephone call in mid-afternoon (when doctors are most under pressure in the office). Realizing that the professions share the trust of their patients, superhuman efforts of patience and cooperation are needed.

Multidisciplinary patient conferences are useful and important. Again, scheduling presents a real problem. The medical coordinator may fill in for the attending physician or conferences can be held early in the morning.

When doctors and nurses recognize professional competence and concern for their patients in their counterparts and are willing to communicate with one another, collaboration can work well, to the patients' benefit.

Clinical Exercises

Frieda Krankenhaus, age 86, has been your family practice patient for many years. Lately, she has both lost capability at independent instrumental activities of daily living and become lonely and isolated at home. A notice arrives in the mail from Finest Hour Retirement Home, announcing that she is about to be admitted to their intermediate care unit. A letter addressed to you from the medical director states that top-quality medical care is expected in the facility and asks you to commit to the following standards:

A yearly history and physical examination on all patients.
Visits every 2 weeks.
A chest x-ray prior to admission.
24-hour availability.
Keeping of all records in the facility.

Are these requests reasonable? Which would you like to discuss with the medical director and possibly change? (Turn to 13.1, page 143.) With the admission material is a form marked "Advance Directives." On it, you are asked to choose for your patient from among four "degrees of intervention"; (1) full cardiac arrest resuscitation and intensive care; (2) hospital admission for acute illness short of intensive care and cardiac arrest resuscitation; (3) treatment for cure in the facility; and (4) treatment for comfort only. There is then a space for your signature at the bottom of the form.

What is your response to this advance directives request? Would you add any other information to the form? (Turn to 13.2, page 143.)

Struggling to see a waiting room full of office patients one afternoon, you receive an apparently urgent call about Mrs. Krankenhaus from a facility nurse. It is 3:30 pm. The nurse has just come on shift, and she has received a written report that Mrs. Krankenhaus has vomited during the day. Would you come and see her please?

Outline your reasonable response to this request. (Turn to 13.3, page 144.)

CHAPTER 14

Palliative Care

Priorities for health care change at the end of life. This is so whether our patients have a specific illness that is expected to be fatal or not. Many frail elderly people require palliative care or care that uses its principles; we hope therefore to be capable at it and to understand it in broad outline.

Palliative care is usually defined as care of dying patients or care directed primarily to comfort rather than cure. One might wonder why we adopt this binary approach, either seeking a diagnosis and striving for a cure or invoking skills and technology to keep someone comfortable. It might seems obvious that very strenuous efforts to achieve comfort are always appropriate, even while we are still hoping to make someone better and to return them to their usual life situation.

Palliative care is perhaps the most humane of medical and other health care. Many of us cannot identify with obstetrical, pediatric, trauma, or system-failure patients, but everyone dies, and so in doing palliative care, it is a bit as though we are looking after ourselves. How best to do this? Fortunately, empathy and caring are enhanced by good technical ability. When we show someone that we understand their problem, can evaluate it capably, and are able to improve things for them, the time we spend in reassurance and counseling is even more effective. The first step in excellent palliative care is determining for ourselves that a painful death or late-life state in someone under our care is never an acceptable situation.

Pain Control

Pain is a consistent preoccupation in palliative care. It is the most common distressing symptom for cancer patients and others beyond cure. Its management should be understood and practiced by everyone doing geriatrics.

Pain is cortically appreciated changes in peripheral sensory receptors. But we understand that it is heavily modified by many things far removed from the receptor itself. *Total pain* means the sensation of hurt or injury, worsened by fear, anger, depression, and other negative states of mind.

That I may die, lose dignity, be humiliated, or suffer dreadful harm to my body are terrifying thoughts. Many illnesses are poorly understood by caregivers, and uncertainty seems to mean the worst for the patient. I may ask myself why there is no bed in the hospital, why my physician is bewildered or ineffective, and why this should all be happening to me. Helplessness makes angry resentment more dreadful and destructive. Abandonment, loss of mastery, and loss of the future may weigh heavily and make me despondent.

The first step in treatment of pain-intensifying states of mind is recognition, followed by sensitive discussion and practical help. Communication may be difficult.

Pain treatment requires objectivity in the face of a subjective problem. Numerical or visual pain scales starting with 0 for no pain and ending with 5 or 10 for the worst pain imaginable can be used for comparison purposes and to help appreciate the severity of a complaint. Variability and incongruity between a numerical report and a predicted pain experience may indicate nonphysiologic factors to be addressed.

Drugs are an indispensable part of pain control. Pharmacokinetics operate to our advantage when we understand them. A sufficient blood level of analgesic drug is necessary for its effectiveness. Therefore, doses must be regular, but they may be augmented with extra medicine for breakthrough pain. Too low a dose permits pain, too high a dose produces sedation. Sedation is no problem at night; pain is a problem at all times. Opioids, the most useful pain medicines, require constipation prevention because of their anticholinergic effects.

Certain opioids are most effective. Codeine, oxycodone, morphine, and hydromorphone are better and longer-acting than meperidine, pentazocine, and propoxyphene. Each drug has a half-life, a starting dose, and a set of adverse

effects. Learning and using this information allows titration (the gradual increase of drug dose to achieve elimination of pain), maintenance (a continuing regimen that keeps
pain under control), and step-up dose increases to cover
worsened pain symptoms.

Many types of pain respond to a narcotic plus another
strategy. A narcotic dose can be reduced, and pain control
improved using these adjuvants. Radiation for isolated
bone tumors, surgery to remove painful masses or relieve
abscesses, nerve blocks, acupuncture, and other techniques
may be helpful.

Co-analgesia is the name given to adjuvant treatment
with drugs. Try the following substances for these specific
pain situations: nonsteroidal anti-inflammatory drugs for
bone or soft tissue pain; corticosteroids for intracranial
pressure nerve compression or hypercalcemia; benzodiazepines for muscle spasm; neuroleptics for tenesmus or anxiety that worsens pain; antidepressants for dysesthesia,
neuralgia, or pain worsened by depression; anticonvulsants for lancinating neuritic pain or for dysesthesia; antiarrhythmic drugs for dysesthesia (mexiletine, flecainide);
antibiotics for cellulitis and infected ulcers; local anesthetics for ulcers and skin breakdown; antispasmodics for
muscle spasms; and nitrous oxide inhaled for short inter-
mittent painful situations.

There is no situation in health care where persistence is
more important than in pain control. The patient will sense
frustration and lack of resolve in the prescriber, and symptoms may be worsened for this reason.

Other Symptoms

Cancer care and symptom control in other serious disease
states requires effective treatment of whatever distresses
the patient. Several recommendations for specific symptom
control are enumerated in the following paragraphs.

For nausea and vomiting, phenothiazines (prochlorperazine, trifluoperazine, or haloperidol) or antihistamines (dimenhydrinate) are traditional drug treatments.
Metoclopromide, domperidone, or cisapride may also be

used to assist in emptying the stomach. Topical scopolamine in a patch behind the ear, corticosteroids, benzodiazepines, and marijuana where allowed, may also be helpful.
Certain foods may not be well tolerated, and a small oral
intake diminishes the sensation of gastric fullness that
leads to some nausea.

Powerful anticholinergic drugs such as atropine, hyoscine, and belladonna–opium combinations may provide
partial relief for even mechanical bowel obstruction. Effective narcotic treatment of pain is essential.

Hiccup may be relieved using chlorpromazine, diazepam,
or phenytoin. Induction of gagging by an object at the back
of the throat may risk producing vomiting, but it can occasionally stop hiccup by relieving gastric distention. Try
rebreathing in a paper bag.

Maintain freedom from constipation with a high-fiber
diet and plenty of fluids, especially in summer. Moderate
constipation responds to irritants (sennosides, for example); stool in rectum can be moved with a suppository or
enema, and an oil-retention enema or large doses of
lactulose may be useful if constipation is severe.

Apparent diarrhea may be fecal impaction and respond to
constipation measures. Otherwise, opium or loperamide
may be necessary and helpful.

Cough may be caused by pressure on the trachea by a
tumor, and chemotherapy or radiation may be helpful. If
bronchospasm is contributing, a salbutamol nebulizer may
be useful. Cough can be suppressed with small doses of
codeine or dextromethorphan.

Patients suffering and frightened with shortness of
breath require a careful medical work-up to define the
cause, for effective symptom relief. Oxygen is rarely useful,
since the cause is usually not hypoxia. Morphine,
neuroleptics, other narcotics, or atropine may improve the
symptoms subjectively. A room with an open window, a fan
by the bedside, and the presence of someone reassuring
may be effective where organic strategies are not.

Care of dying and very ill patients directed toward symptom control is wonderfully rewarding to practice. If, for any
reason, you are not comfortable with this type of work,
consider a little extra training to improve your confidence.

Recognize, though, that excellent palliative care is an absolute necessity and a basic minimum acceptable standard of care. The choice, then, is not between excellent and adequate palliative care but between excellent palliative care, which you do yourself, and that done by someone else accustomed to providing it. The time will come for most of us when that standard will personally serve us well.

Clinical Exercises

Maria Crabbe, age 77, has known metastatic breast cancer. You are asked to undertake her primary medical care since her previous family physician does not make house calls.

On the first visit, she describes quite severe mid-thoracic back pain that is keeping her awake at night. The pain was well-controlled in the hospital with injections; she now has tablets, which you identify as pentazocine 30 mg, that she takes every few hours when the pain is severe. The medication is only partly effective. The pain is worsened by movement, not related to any bodily functions, and has been worsening slowly. She has no problem with her bowels and is otherwise feeling fine so far. What action could you take initially to help her?

1. Increase the pentazocine to 2 tabs q4h around the clock (turn to 14.1, page 144).
2. Substitute controlled-release morphine 15 mg po bid (turn to 14.2, page 144).
3. Substitute controlled-release morphine 15 mg po bid and provide a nonsustained-release morphine liquid to be given 5–10 mg q4h as required for breakthrough pain (turn to 14.3, page 145).
4. Perform a careful physical examination of the chest, abdomen, and thoracic spine (turn to 14.4, page 145).

Thoracic spine physical examination reveals some quite marked superficial musculoskeletal tenderness at about the level of T6 to the right of the spine. An injection of lidocaine at the painful focus produces marked pain relief, although there is a second thoracic back pain, lower down, which persists. You follow the lidocaine with an injection of corticosteroid and find that partial pain relief is eventually sustained. Moderate doses of codeine are sufficient to control the remaining pain.

Months later, on higher doses of narcotic for pain, Mrs. Crabbe is losing weight and having trouble maintaining hydration due to nausea and vomiting. Physical examination shows some evidence of immobile masses in the midabdomen, but there is no evidence of bowel obstruction. What do you suggest at this stage?

1. Dimenhydrinate 50 mg po q4h prn nausea (turn to 14.5, page 145).
2. Prochlorperazine 10 mg po tid (turn to 14.6, page 145).
3. Metoclopramide 10 mg po tid (turn to 14.7, page 146).
4. Restrict oral intake (turn to 14.8, page 146)

CHAPTER 15

Ethical Issues

Giving health care to others places us in special situations not always addressed by our formal professional training. Sometimes we confront an apparent "no-win" choice and are expected to do difficult, even morally questionable, things such as take risks, withhold the truth, withhold "textbook" care, or disregard a statement of preference to do our jobs properly.

Ethics is the branch of philosophy that deals with moral judgment, which we health professionals exercise daily. In this chapter, we explore three areas of health care that are controversial and where moral judgment is necessary: euthanasia, or mercy killing; capability (people's ability to make decisions and understand complicated questions); and the making of decisions for people who are not capable.

Euthanasia

Death is awful, and inevitable. It is understandable that we want to try to postpone it or attempt to improve its often very unpleasant circumstances. Is anything worse than death? Most of us surmise that prolonged severe or extreme mental or physical pain might qualify. If this were the case, it could occur that someone would wish to die to end a situation worse than death. As professionals, we may need to consider permitting, assisting with, or causing someone's death in such a situation.

There is a heirarchy of euthanasia. If we do not provide theoretically curative care that is obviously futile in a practical setting, especially if our patient has requested us to refrain, most people would agree we are acting properly. Once having started a course of treatment, it is generally held to be appropriate to stop it if it becomes futile. When experienced professionals, patients' close relatives and loved ones, and various administrative and legal authorities are in agreement with us in these actions, we feel more secure about them and are probably less likely to regret them.

Controversy surrounds assisted suicide. This "voluntary active euthanasia" may seem to support someone's autonomy, as they request our assistance in dying. It can be argued that there is no moral difference between taking action and refraining from action if the outcome, death, is the same. We may see not assisting with a suicide as active prolonging of suffering, which is probably morally intolerable.

On the other hand, entire religious traditions in many societies hold that death is God's business, not people's. A profession that agrees to assist with death is arguably functioning as a sort of executioner and may be in conflict with its ethical standards if they include saving or maintaining life.

Voluntary active euthanasia is a theoretical question for most of us, since we work in countries where it is illegal, and we would not wish to break the law. It is left to us simply to be very good indeed at symptom control, certainly a more traditional role for health care providers. The controversy will continue, and assisted suicide is a matter to wrestle with in one's conscience.

Active non-voluntary euthanasia and involuntary active euthanasia are "mercy killing" of incompetent people, and killing against someone's will. The moral dangers of doing away with people unable to make decisions because we believe their lives to be intolerable are quite significant. It might be difficult to be sure how intolerable someone's subjective experience is, and one might be tempted to mercy killing for reasons perhaps less than merciful. Killing someone against their will is appropriately punishable as murder.

Capability

Human activity is inescapably mental. Some of our more important actions, including making a will, managing money, marrying, and consenting to treatment, require us to understand what we are doing and to make decisions. But what if we or someone for whom we have responsibility cannot understand or decide?

Capability and guardianship laws are being reformed in many places. Health professionals need to be familiar with what the law says about these matters before making judgments and pronouncements about them.

Asked to evaluate someone's capability, we are most successful when we observe certain rules. Capability must be presumed until clear proof indicates otherwise. It is very important to tell someone that their capability is at issue before evaluating it. Capability is never global but applies to a particular task, and it can only be stated for the particular time at which it was evaluated. Someone who, on Thursday, can understand how much money they have and to whom they wish to leave it when they die, may still be incapable of the details of managing that money or less understanding on the next Sunday. Tests of cognition (Chapter 6) and a thorough mental status examination proceed to psychiatric or neurobehavioral diagnoses. These measurements and conclusions are valuable in understanding capability, but they are only part of the story; there is no Mini-Mental Status Examination score that always corresponds to capability for specific tasks. The standard of capability required to deal with small financial matters and to make low-risk care decisions is less than that needed for very large amounts of money and grave risks.

Specific questions are used to evaluate ability to do a specific task. After a discussion of the possible outcomes of a course of treatment, the patient may be asked to describe the best- and worst-case scenarios if they decide for or against being treated. Arithmetic and financial questions pertain to financial capability. The answers to questions about someone's finances may seem reasonable and yet be incorrect, so they require confirmation by some other reliable person.

Your documentation of capability evaluations is extremely important because a lot may depend on your being able to demonstrate objectively that your conclusions are reasonable. Remember when making notes that someone may be reading or listening to your opinion in a critical way in the future.

Very difficult and impossible situations arise in capability evaluation, and you may need help, require other evaluation, or be unable to reach a conclusion. Don't be afraid to take the appropriate action in these situations, even if it includes stating that no conclusion can be reached.

Deciding for Incompetent People

If you conclude that someone is unable to give you instructions for their care, you must find another way to make decisions for them. This is the reason for advance directives. You are in the best position to make a quality decision for someone if you know what they might have wanted in the past, when they were capable of a reasonable decision.

If no autonomous decision (one made by a capable person at the time in question about the matter at issue) is available, there may have been a previous decision on the issue. This would be a "living will" or equivalent, which specifies what to do in a particular situation. If there is no previous decision, the person may have delegated someone to assist in making decisions when they are incapable. This substituted decision-maker would then function as though they were the patient themselves and decide. If neither previous decision nor a substitute decision-maker is available, a gathering of information, including the opinions of everyone involved in caregiving and close to the person, is necessary, and an understanding must be reached about that person's known opinions on similar matters, religious and ideological views, and feelings about life in general. You are then in a position to make a decision that you believe would be in that person's best interest.

Choosing the most morally right option in a difficult situation can be very challenging. These few guidelines may be helpful in some situations; an ability to think logically and humanely about ethical issues is something every health professional should work at developing.

Clinical Exercises

Here, we offer two scenarios for your consideration. Unlike the other chapters, no "correct" answers are provided.

Case 1

An elderly woman with known cancer of the bowel has been admitted to the hospital for terminal pain control. She was managed at home with the assistance of sympathetic and knowledgeable relatives, using a portable parenteral narcotic pump. This had been effective, but fecal incontinence, along with confusion, has made home care more than the family can tolerate.

The confusion may be due to narcotic (she was using hydromorphone 40 mg q2h by pump), but you believe it is mainly caused by central nervous system metastases, since she remained confused when the pump was temporarily not functioning.

On the second hospital day, you arrive in the morning and find that pain control has not been adequate through the night, in spite of increasing doses of parenteral narcotic. The patient is uncomfortable, constantly moaning and clutching at her pelvis. Nursing reports two periods of near apnea during the night as well.

You are asked whether further narcotic dose increases would be appropriate, given that respiratory depression is obviously occurring. What are your orders?

Case 2

A man recently admitted to an intermediate care facility requires advance directives according to the facility guidelines.

You sit down with him to discuss cardiac arrest resuscitation. He does not understand what the term means, and so you explain that if the heart stops beating, it is possible to attempt to restart it by blows, electric shock, and drugs. He states that yes, of course, he would want that done if it might restart his heart. You then explain that these measures are effective only 20% of the time, and that elderly people whose heartbeat is restarted only very rarely survive intact; more often, they have worsened brain damage and poor quality of life following the resuscitation.

He then says that he still would wish the resuscitation to be attempted, since if the outcome were poor, the caregivers could then simply "let him go," and he would die peacefully. You explain that, once resuscitated it is far from certain that someone will go on to expire in a short time. He says that this is not important, he still feels the same way.

Does this man understand the circumstances well enough to have his wishes followed? Under what circumstances would you oppose his wishes? If you believed him incompetent to make this decision, what options would be open to you?

Responses to Clinical Exercises

1.1

Although it is speculative, we feel this is the most limited of the aging theories. It seems that there must be both an evolutionary dimension as well as an environmental one to explain the slow destruction we call aging.

1.2

Destructive forces undoubtedly contribute to tissue deterioration that aggregates into aging, but biology is full of organisms and living structures that constantly survey and repair themselves. Why don't we? (see 1.3, following)

1.3

If chickens in the wild over eons are consumed by predators at an average age of 12 weeks, and none survive beyond 20 weeks, a cellular repair mechanism that maintained chicken tissue intact beyond, say, 16 weeks would not survive in large numbers to subsequent generations. In other words, it would not be selected. The same may be true of potential repair mechanisms that could allow humans to maintain intact body tissues indefinitely.

2.1

This response looks as though you are (at best) keen on evaluating the diabetes, heart disease, and possible furosemide side effects, and (at worst) can't wait to get this problem out of the office. Principles of comprehensive geriatric assessment suggest that you will need more and different information to get a handle on this lady's situation. Reread the chapter (page 11) or look over the notes (page 152), and then carry on with question 2 on page 20.

2.2

The physical exam would naturally follow the history. Diabetes and heart disease are not a bad place to start, but there is some more, and more likely valuable, information to be obtained first. Frequent calls for help may reflect confusion, real requirement for assistance, or both. How "with it" is she? How independent? Look over the notes on comprehensive geriatric assessment (page 152), and then carry on with the next part of this case (page 20).

2.3

This is one of two acceptable answers here. An ill-defined and caregiving-centered presenting complaint is very common in the frail elderly, but the problem will often involve a mental or physical disability leading to collapse of independence. You will get hints about mental capability and coping ability with the questions asked in this choice. You could also get your answers with direct questioning and testing. Take a look at item III, page 152, in the notes on comprehensive geriatric assessment. Then proceed with the next question on this case (page 21).

2.4

Quite right. This specific information will take you to the heart of the matter in this apparently frail older woman. Is she telephoning out of forgetfulness and bewilderment, has a capability deterioration exposed basic ADL needs, or both? With this information, you're in a position to direct your further history and physical. Turn to page 21 to continue with this case.

2.5

We hope you included some or all of the following:

Is she taking her medication and how do we know?
Does she drink alcohol?
Has she had psychological problems in the past?
How is she getting around? Any falls?
In this new troubled situation, who is taking responsibility
   for her?
Does she drive a car? Any suggestion of a near-fire?
Is she incontinent of bowels or urine?

If your list included five, congratulations. Carry on with
the case on page 21. If you got two to four, take a look at IV-
B in the notes (page 155). If you got only one or zero, reread
the chapter on comprehensive geriatric assessment and
consider some memorizing of the notes. Then on with the
case, page 21.

2.6

We would act promptly to attempt to address the following:

The delirium
The hyperthyroidism
The medication compliance problems and possible overuse
   or underuse

We feel that secondary, potentially significant priorities
would include:

The cataracts
The incontinence
The back pain and knee osteoarthritis

Ultimately, it looks as though this is a delirium due to
hyperthyroidism, probably superimposed on an early
dementia. Previous level of function was apparently not
bad, but supports may be required. If you focused on the
hyperthyroidism and the medication, and understood their
possible roles in delirium, carry on to Chapter 3. If you
missed them or tended to take an interest in other "red

herring" problem list items, consider taking another look at Chapter 2 before proceeding.

3.1

This appears to have been the admitting diagnosis, and angina and congestive heart failure have been treated with the heavy-handed characteristic of someone determined to eradicate them. Still, there was no myocardial infarct, your physical examination does not confirm continuing disabling congestive heart failure, and chest pain is not a major complaint. Something else may be going on here. Since this is the chapter on medication, you may want to look over it (page 23) or its notes (page 157) again to sharpen your instincts. Please read 3.4, following, and then return to page 30.

3.2

He is on antibiotics, was seen by an infectious diseases specialist, and is tachypneic, but he has been discharged and appears to have had a steadily improving hospital course. Survival of bacteria in the atmosphere of his antibiotic regime is difficult to imagine. Have a look at the notes on prescribing for the elderly (page 157), then read 3.4, following.

3.3

Neurology did see him in the hospital, but we don't find evidence of them having found parkinsonism (ie, anti-Parkinson's medication). There are signs of parkinsonism, which may be new, especially if the daughter's history of previous good mobility is accurate. He is also on a lot of loxapine. But we still have the rapid respiratory rate, hypotension, and confusion to account for, as well as the postural unsteadiness. Parkinson's may be present, but it's probably not what is really slowing him down. Read the notes on prescribing for the elderly (page 157), and then read 3.4, following.

3.4

This is an awful lot of medication, isn't it? Many unpleasant things could have happened to this man in the hospital, necessitating the multiple subspeciality consultations and causing him to need all these drugs. In our experience, however (and possibly also in yours), drugs are more often part of the problem than part of the solution. Given a field of patients like this one, more than half will be suffering remediable adverse drug reactions (those from medications that could be stopped). Carry on with the case on page 30.

3.5

Omeprazole's main offense is its cost. It is a stunningly effective acid suppressor that has few adverse consequences in the elderly. It may be unnecessary, but it is probably also innocuous. It's the worst choice of the four; perhaps a reread of Chapter 3 would help you.

3.6

Although loxapine is not a bad choice for agitation in the elderly, 5 mg three times a day is very heavy handed. This drug came from the neurologist, who was called to the coronary care unit (CCU) because of confusion. Unable to get collateral history, he presumed dementia and acted to control the delirium, which he also recognized was present. Unfortunately, released to the open ward, Mr. Doperman had his loxapine continued. He now suffers mobility problems, part of the hypotension, and some blunting of his cognitive capacity from this medication. We feel it is the most important one to stop, probably in three fairly quick increments. Carry on with Chapter 4.

3.7

Enalapril works well for congestive heart failure. Unfortunately, it can also depress blood pressure, worsen renal failure, and increase potassium. You may have detected an absence of congestive heart failure signs here and the presence of a low blood pressure. We agree enalapril would be a good candidate for reduction but suspect that the delirium this man is suffering is based more on loxapine. It is important to reduce one drug at a time, and loxapine would be our first choice.

3.8

There is no rationale for sotalol based on the information we have. If you discontinue it, arrhythmia or angina might rebound, but the unexplained tachypnea could improve if there is reversible airway disease, and the blood pressure will certainly get a bit better. Beta blockers are often harmful in older people for these and other reasons. We would choose sotalol as the second most important drug to stop here, after loxapine, which is contributing to parkinsonism and delirium. Carry on with Chapter 4.

4.1

People can certainly fall if their cardiac output changes suddenly. This is, however, neither a very common cause of falling nor a frequently rewarding one to search for, in spite of its being "high profile" and easy to diagnose. Holter monitors are often negative or show arrhythmias that didn't really cause the fall. Read over "Remediable Mobility Failure Causes," page 35 before continuing with the case, page 38.

The most common cause of falls in the elderly is, like the most common cause of almost every symptom or presentation, multiple causes.

4.2

This is a good answer, since drugs often contribute to falling through orthostatic hypotension and an altered state of consciousness. The most common cause of falls is, however, multiple causes (also the most common cause of nearly every other presentation or symptom in older people). Carry on with this case on page 38.

4.3

Correct. The most common cause of *any* presentation or symptom in older people tends to be multiple causes. Falling represents failure of a complex interaction of psychological and biological functions, and aging affects them all. The important question is which, if any, are remediable. Carry on with the case on page 38.

4.4

Problems in the home environment, including loose carpets, dark stairways, and slippery floors, are very important causes of falling and are often overlooked by physicians since they are not "medical." They most often, however, contribute to falls in an already-compromised individual, in other words, someone with multiple falling causes. This is the most common cause of falls and of a great many other things in older people. Carry on with the case on page 38.

4.5

Medication (there is no congestive heart failure and certainly no hypertension to justify the captopril).

Any fainting cause (vasovagal syncope, arrhythmia, TIA, or drop attack may be involved).

Recent illness (the findings are subtle, but the decreased air entry and hypothermia may indicate an occult pneumonia).

Environmental hazards (someone needs to have a look at that apartment).

Mechanical foot problems.

Gait or balance disturbance (this has not yet been specifically evaluated).

4.6

If you chose this answer, you do need to read the chapter on mobility failure or read it again with better comprehension. A traditional static neurological examination tells us very little about gait and balance. Acquaint yourself with the other means of evaluating this before continuing to the next chapter.

4.7

This is a quite acceptable way of evaluating gait, but you may miss problems with static balance. Safety can be evaluated by simple observed walking, and lack of dynamic (walking) balance picked up. A specific gait disturbance may point to a diagnosis. Standing still, however, may reveal problems not apparent while moving. If you are not already familiar with the "get up and go" test, quickly read over "The Specific Mobility Evaluation," page 34, before proceeding to the next chapter.

4.8

This is the means we recommend for obtaining static and dynamic balance and gait evaluation in a reproducible way. Once you know how to do the test, proceed to the next chapter.

5.1

This sort of first step will keep nobody but pharmaceutical company representatives happy. Although the history rules out a few remediable incontinence causes, others are lying well up the list from a trial of anticholinergics. Read Chapter 5 again, and then go on to Case 2, page 45.

5.2

Ruling out obstruction is a wise and necessary step. You may even obtain a specimen with your catheter sample to pick off urinary tract infection as a possible remediable cause. This maneuver, although it is an acceptable answer, would ordinarily follow culture and rectal examination to rule out fecal impaction. Carry on with Case 2, page 45.

5.3

You have chosen the next step in the algorithm; congratulations. A positive culture does not guarantee a remediable cause, but a trial of therapy is necessary. Although fecal impaction is unlikely to be the only cause in this chronic incontinence, it is worth ruling out and cleaning up. Carry on with Case 2, page 45.

5.4

Not quite. Even in a chronically incontinent chairfast man, there may be enough cognition and expressive ability to call for the bottle when the bladder is full. Take another look at the algorithm for incontinence evaluation (Figure 5.2) page 42, and then proceed with Case 2 (page 45).

5.5

Flavoxate is not, last time we looked, a first-line drug for the management of incontinence at this lady's stage of investigation. She may yet have a contribution from pure stress incontinence, atrophic urethritis, or detrusor instability. Take a look at the algorithm (Figure 5.2) on page 42, and perhaps reread Chapter 5 if you have time. Then carry on with Chapter 6.

5.6

This simple measure would probably help a great deal. There are still a few remediable medical conditions to be considered and ruled out, however, which are shown in the algorithm (Figure 5.2) on page 42. Once you understand these, carry on with Chapter 6.

5.7

A trial of estrogen at this stage is not a bad idea. If she responds, it can be continued (assuming no contraindications); if she doesn't, less innocuous measures can be tried, such as referral for bladder suspension (after appropriate investigation) and trial of anticholinergics. On to Chapter 6.

5.8

This is a tricky answer to evaluate. It could be a good move if your consultant recognizes that everyone with a stress incontinence symptom does not necessarily benefit from a stress incontinence procedure and does some urodynamic evaluation. If not, you could be sending your patient for useless and risky surgery. Look over the last leg of the algorithm (Figure 5.2) on page 42 before proceeding to Chapter 6.

6.1

To be systematic, this is the best answer of the four choices, although all the others are important as well. This is a difficult clinical problem with a number of worrisome possibilities, but well done for focusing on the issue that will help you to think clearly about confusion. Carry on to the next step in this case, back on page 52.

6.2

This man may have psychological symptoms, since he is reported as confused. If he had been a psychiatric patient in the past, it would be useful to know. On the other hand, systematic confusion evaluation requires an understanding of the presence or absence of cognitive impairment and just how bad it is as a first step. Psychiatric patients also develop delerium. Take a look at "Confusion Triage," page 46, before proceeding with the rest of the case on page 52.

6.3

This may be a very important issue. If you chose it as the first priority here, it is hard to fault your judgment. We are encouraging a systematic approach to cognitive impairment triage, however, and (although you may need to understand the language issue to find out) the first problem is whether this man is cognitively impaired or not. If you understood that first priority, carry on with this case on page 52. Otherwise, review the cognitive impairment triage diagram on page 47.

6.4

Hypotension and confusion in a postoperative patient raises several medical concerns, one of them infection. None of the answers you could have chosen here is entirely wrong, but this is perhaps the worst of the four, since it appears to bypass some important steps in a systematic approach to the confused patient. This man will need a careful medical evaluation in the next short while, but the presentation is that of confusion, and the first step is to determine what his cognitive status is. Please review the cognitive impairment triage diagram on page 47, before continuing with the case back on page 52.

6.5

Yes, he is cognitively impaired, unless there is an unrecognized problem with the interpretation process. On the issue of delirium, it is hard to judge from the information provided. Attention is not yet evaluated, really. There is a cognitive change, the time course is unknown, and a recent postop patient is certainly in a classic delirium-producing situation. Yet he focuses on and answers the questions, although incorrectly. Review the section on delirium, page 48, before reading the denouement on page 53.

6.6

There is enough detail in this history to convince most people that the message is getting past the language barrier but that the answers coming back are tending to be incorrect. A few correct answers indicate intact communication, and so cognitive impairment is almost certainly present. Look over confusion triage, page 46, before reading what finally happened on page 53.

6.7

This is a difficult case and a somewhat artificial one, which doesn't make it any easier. It is also true that there is a "curtain" of attention deficiency in delirium, which may preclude accurate cognitive impairment evaluation. This man, however, looks cognitively impaired by his incorrect answers and near misses, but he has not yet given us convincing evidence of a disorder of attention. We may infer delirium from the setting, but the evidence is thin so far. Please review the delirium criteria on page 48 and then read what happens on page 53.

6.8

This is the most correct of the four answers. He gets orientation and memory questions wrong, but not entirely wrong. This indicates that he is capable of paying attention, but that he has deficiencies in higher mental functioning. In other words, he is cognitively impaired. His attention to questions sounds adequate, but has not been specifically evaluated. Therefore, although a postoperative patient may easily be delirious for a number of reasons, no conclusion can be drawn yet about delirium. Find out what happens by reading the last paragraph on page 53.

7.1

Well, she is anhedonic, but she denies dysphoria, has no sleep disorder, guilt, or thought problems, and she denies suicide. Her energy is poor, there is some history of weight loss, and the psychomotor rate is hard to evaluate. You could be right, or you could be wrong: but will it help with her care? If you know and use the DSM-IV criteria and recognize their limitations in the elderly, proceed to the next step in this case, page 60. If you were guessing, look at the criteria summary on page 170 or (better yet) read the chapter again.

7.2

See 7.1.

7.3

You correctly focus on the limitations of DSM-IV criteria in depression diagnosis in the elderly. But irrelevant? Probably not quite. This lady is borderline in terms of her major depressive episode, but she has other suggestive features to her presentation such as a global failure to thrive and a positive functional inquiry with a negative physical examination. The DSM-IV criteria are a starting point, and in this case we are led to suspect depression strongly but cannot confirm the diagnosis. Reread the first part of the chapter and then continue with this case on page 60.

7.4

A major depressive episode should involve depression not due to the effects of a substance. Propranolol can cause depression, and it may be part of the problem here. Unless it was started just before she began to deteriorate, however, it is unlikely to be the whole story. Carry on with the case on page 60.

7.5

Some geriatric psychiatrists currently recommend this as a first-choice drug in selected elderly people with depression. We believe, at this stage, that primary care doctors should still be using straight serotonin or noradrenalin-influencing medication as a first line, however. Sertraline, paroxetine, or fluvoxamine might be acceptable choices. Nortryptiline would be less so, because of the orthostatic hypotension. Reread "Treatment of Depression," page 58, before continuing with Chapter 8.

7.6

Of the four possibilities, this seems the safest and likely most effective choice. You apparently recognize that ortho-static hypotension is a relative contraindication to nortryptiline and that fluoxetine causes problems in the elderly. Carry on with Chapter 8.

7.7

Bad choice. Fluoxetine was effective and less harmful than some tricyclics in the few years when it was the only sero-tonin reuptake inhibitor available. There are now safer drugs, which do not have as long half-lives and which cause less agitation, weight loss, and movement disorder. Have another look at "Treatment of Depression," page 58, before carrying on with Chapter 8.

7.8

Well, this would not have been a bad choice in the late 1980s, even in the face of this patient's orthostatic hypotension. Today, there are safer medications in this situation. Read over "Treatment of Depression," page 58, before proceeding. Some specialists still use nortryptiline before selective serotonin reuptake inhibitors (SSRI), but orthostatic hypotension would clinch its riskiness here for the majority.

8.1

This action indicates alarm at a dangerous situation. It might be appropriate if the son had threatened escalating physical violence, especially if the mother were not as de-pendent on him. As it is, you might risk the authorities' feeling obliged to remove the patient from a perceived dan-ger, which could result in unwanted facility placement. Quickly reread the latter part of the section on elder abuse, page 61, before proceeding to the next case, page 67.

8.2

This seems the strategy most likely to achieve the best of all worlds here, in which the caregiving situation is preserved and the abuse ceases. If the son, in your judgment, is dangerous and violent, the authorities can then be notified. If he has concerns potentially amenable to talking-out, this can be tried. Carry on with the next case, page 67.

8.3

We do see a need for action here. Although your patient's life and safety are probably not in immediate danger, the situation is deteriorating and appears to need some intervention. We would call the son in for a friendly chat and proceed as indicated based on his response to being confronted. Look over the section on elder abuse, page 61, before proceeding to the next case, page 67.

8.4

Some psychologists are excellent at evaluating and intervening with abuse. Our experience suggests that more time and expense than might readily be available here could be consumed in this process. Why not have a frank chat with the son yourself and see how dangerous you believe he is? This is probably a reasonable and safe option, however, if you aren't comfortable with awkward psychosocial issues yourself, or if the counsellor you have in mind is especially effective. Turn to the next case, page 67.

8.5

Respecting the confidence in the home care nurse is important. This strategy of linking to alcohol symptoms identified by the patient as unpleasant and disabling sometimes works. Direct confrontation and an unrealistic expectation of abstinence, on the other hand, are rarely effective in the elderly. Carry on with the next case, page 68.

8.6

Support group, complete abstinence, and "cards on the table" confrontation tend to be catastrophic in the elderly, although they often work in younger adults. This lady is frail, her independence is fragile, and the extent of her drinking problem is not known. Approach with caution. Take another look at the section on alcohol, page 63, before proceeding with the third case, page 68.

8.7

This, like using Alcoholics Anonymous, is often a maneuver doomed to failure in frail elderly. She will lose confidence in the home care nurse and instinctively recognize you as an unrealistic enemy whose advice, if followed, will destroy her independence. She is right. Read over the section on alcohol, page 63, before proceeding with the next case, page 68.

8.8

Spoken like a true old-fashioned office internist. We trust your reading the response to this answer doesn't indicate a serious intention to chose it over the others. This woman requires sensitive and knowledgeable handling in the psychosocial sphere. Her physical problems are significant, but discovering a gastritis and treating it with omeprazole will not solve her problems. Read the section on alcohol, page 63, before looking over the next case, page 68.

8.9

Ageism! There are people who should not be driving at 35 and others who are still safe approaching 100. It is this man's hand deformity and mild cognitive impairment that could cause driving problems. Please read the section on driving, page 64, before proceeding to Chapter 9. We would road test this man.

8.10

Cognitive impairment and driving are a real problem. Our current practice is to restrict driving when memory and orientation problems begin to interfere with judgment. This is difficult to measure, except by direct evaluation. We suggest a road test here. His Folstein score of 26 is not incompatible with driving, although some restrictions of speed, night driving, and geographical range might be appropriate. Frequent reevaluation of cognition would be necessary. Have another look at the section on driving, page 64, before proceeding with Chapter 9.

8.11

Contraindications there aren't, but we see a couple of caution flashers here in the hand deformity and early cognitive impairment. Road test and careful reevaluation every 6 months or so seem prudent. Check the section on driving, page 64, once more before proceeding with Chapter 9.

8.12

This is our usual practice when in doubt about a driver's ability. His cognitive impairment is not bad enough to prohibit him by itself, he may compensate for the hand deformity, and age alone is no indication of safety. Continue with Chapter 9.

9.1

You can never go wrong increasing the bulk in someone's diet, although we wonder sometimes how valuable still more bran, prunes, etc. will be in someone already eating fiber with every meal. This is an acceptable answer, although modifying her medication (which appears in part not to be necessary) would have been our first choice. Carry on with Case 2, page 76.

9.2

This is the comic relief answer here; if you seriously chose it, you need more than just a reread of Chapter 9, which, however, we strongly recommend. A common-sense approach to this problem will solve it 98% of the time. If it fails, then comes the time for medical pyrotechnics. Case studies continue on page 76.

9.3

The laxative regime is actually step 3 in our method of handling apparent functional constipation. Remember that many or most functional constipation problems are amenable to lowering expectations, stopping harmful medication, and diet/hydration/mobility modification. Read the Chapter 9 summary, page 177 over once more before continuing the case studies, page 76.

9.4

This would indeed be our choice for an appropriate first step. Although it might not be the only constipation cause, evidence of uncontrolled congestive heart failure is lacking here, and she may be overdoing the codeine. Diet, hydration, and mobility would follow, and then a sensible laxative regimen, if necessary. Carry on with the next case study, page 76.

9.5

This is a reasonable next step. Since this man appears not to have responded to a bowel clean-out strategy, he may have a diarrhea cause or local anal or rectal abnormality. He has been in acute care and subject to our friends in Infectious Diseases, however, and antibiotic-associated diarrhea (sometimes caused by C. *difficile*) may be part of the problem. Congratulations for following the protocol. Continue with Case 3, page 76.

9.6

This may be effective symptom control, but you appear to neglect the possibility of diarrhea causes that may be remediable. Review the protocol for fecal impaction, page 73, before proceeding with Case 3.

9.7

Instinct and familiarity with the circumstances suggest to you, correctly, that this man's problem may be antibiotic associated. A trial of metronidazole is reasonable, even without waiting for the results of the toxin assay. Carry on with Case 3, page 76.

9.8

Unfortunately, regularizing measures are not normally helpful unless a bowel clean out has been successful. Success means that the fecal incontinence stops, at least temporarily. A search for diarrhea causes (especially considering he has been exposed to antibiotics recently) may be rewarding. Please review fecal incontinence, page 73, before proceeding with Case 3, page 76.

9.9

Nursing time is at a tremendous premium. Q 4 hourly may not be quite frequent enough to avoid all pressure in this patient, but, if she is lying on her side, it is likely sufficient. There are more practical steps to be taken here (debridement, more rational wound treatment, and improvement of general health, for example). Read over the notes on wound care, page 178 before carrying on with Chapter 10.

9.10

This would be one of our top three choices for certain. Carry on with Chapter 10, page 78.

9.11

Strong chemicals belong in the broom closet. Good old 1/4 strength Dakin's is bad enough; increasing this caustic brew will only burn out any remaining granulation tissue. Better have another look at the end of Chapter 9 before proceeding with Chapter 10.

9.12

Infectious disease academic wisdom to the contrary, we find there is little advantage in practice to culturing pressure sores, especially when local conditions do not indicate infection. Check the last part of Chapter 9 before proceeding to Chapter 10.

9.13

We agree that strong chemicals have no place in modern wound care. If you also chose debridement and 9.14, proceed with Chapter 10.

9.14

Possibly you won't help much by improving the nutritional status of this slowly healing tissue. On the other hand, nothing ventured, nothing gained. We agree this would be one of the three choices. Carry on with Chapter 10.

10.1

Many remediable causes of agitation can be uncovered by a good physical examination, including mental status examination and a laboratory work-up. This is indispensable, but on balance, we would probably attempt symptomatic treatment of this very difficult man, first, both to make physical examination possible and to demonstrate to facility staff that immediate transfer to a special unit may not be necessary. Take a quick look at "Approaches to Treatment" in the summary of Chapter 10, page 181, before returning to page 84 to finish this case.

10.2

This is the choice we would favor. Theoretically, treating remediable causes of agitation is a first priority, but in this situation symptomatic treatment is necessary both to proceed with investigation and to prevent facility staff from an unnecessary subspecialist evaluation before your primary care work is done. (Turn to page 84 to continue with the case).

10.3

A behavioral approach to agitation control should never be overlooked. We intended, in this case, to impress you with the need for more biological action. Clinical experience suggest that symptomatic treatment and physical evaluation are the first priorities here. Have another look at the summary of the chapter on difficult behavior, page 180 before returning to page 84, to continue the case.

10.4

Delirium may be part of the problem here, granted; head injury and stroke are possible causes, as well. Acute functional psychiatric disturbance can also precipitate the kind of behavior we see here. But in choosing this answer, we think you're barking up the wrong tree since more conveniently accessible delirium causes may exist, and this very severe agitation requires symptomatic control before any investigation and care can proceed. Look again at the chapter on difficult behavior, page 78, and then turn to page 84, to continue with the case.

10.5

We think you missed the point. Orthostatic hypotension, tachycardia, hyponatremia, and azotemia in the absence of congestive heart failure suggests delirium due to too much furosemide. Monitoring is essential, of course, but there is a remediable cause here, potentially. Please review the summary of the chapter on difficult behavior, page 180, before returning to page 84 to finish this case.

10.6

He is azotemic, but there is a much more obvious and common cause than obstruction, especially since he is continuing to pass water. Volume depletion, evident on physical examination, is probably contributing to the agitation, as well. Once this is corrected, if the creatinine did not fall, ultrasound might be indicated. We would stop the furosemide and see what happens. Although you may benefit from a reread of the material on difficult behavior, seriously choosing this answer suggests that clinical experience will help you more. Turn to page 85 to see the end of this case.

10.7

Correct, of course. Is there really (was there ever) any congestive heart failure here? You could review the hospital admission records, but this judicious trial of therapy is a more reliable way of answering the question. If, as you suspect, delirium due to dehydration is part of the problem, the behavior will improve along with the volume. If not, you can look further. Read the case's completion on page 85.

10.8

The physical examination strongly suggests dehydration, and a prime delirium candidate of that kind shouldn't have escaped your notice. We find prn neuroleptics a poor idea in agitation control, since nurses who decide on drug administration have varying thresholds for dosing, and neuroleptics may require days to reach a steady state. A prn loxapine appears to us to be closing the barn door after the horse has departed, in many cases. Remember that delirium causes reversible agitation. Proceed to the end of this case on page 85.

11.1

A Clinical nurse and a social worker are normally two other essential roles. Budget permitting, rehabilitation professionals, a pharmacist, a nutritionist, and perhaps a neuropsychologist would be helpful. These individuals may be added part-time or used on a case-consulted basis from the community. Read over the summary of Chapter 11 (page 183), if you didn't get the answers on this one. Otherwise, turn back to page 93, and continue.

11.2

As clients are evaluated, someone must keep track of their problems and any progress made in solving them. This role is called *case management*, and it can be accomplished by any of the core professionals. Patients can be delegated to each professional to case-manage sequentially, thus spreading the load. Case managers should be full-time. If, for example, the physician is not in the program at all times, case management might be difficult for him or her. Continue with the questions on page 93.

11.3

1. Client identification and screening.
2. Intake evaluation (comprehensive geriatric assessment).
3. Planning conference (problems identified and responsibility assigned).
4. Designate case manager.
5. Multidisciplinary assessment.
6. Progress conference.
7. Separation.

If you had this sequence pretty well complete or something similar to it, congratulations. If not, take another look at

Chapter 11 or review the outline on page 183, and carry on with the exercise on page 93.

11.4

Reporting and responsibility should be clear. If the director hires and evaluates the other unit members, everyone should understand this. If there is a rule about client attendance and continuation in the program, it should be clear as well. Finally, overlapping of roles needs to be checked out and responsibility defined. A frank talk between the clinical nurse and unit director might make all the difference. Carry on with Chapter 12.

12.1

Most home care programs emphasize management of acute illness at home. Problems associated with hospital admission, including enforced immobility and loss of dignity, might be avoided. Home is a familiar environment and existing social contacts are maintained. The facility would be an unknown and a step that might be difficult to retrace. If the home care service is good and willing in-house medical care is available, an institution may be unnecessary and care quality may be as good at home. Please turn back to page 99, for more questions on home care.

12.2

You will have to share clinical decision-making with other team members. The leadership or case management role must be negotiated, and you may have to relinquish some clinical autonomy. Seeing patients at home imposes time and convenience constraints. If you are the primary care physician and on-call arrangements are not in place, you may have to visit at home (not transfer to the emergency room) in a sudden change in health status. Transfer to the hospital for admission may be limited, if it is your habit frequently to evaluate patients there. Multidisciplinary conferences may be difficult to schedule and require some of your time. You must maintain careful surveillance of your patient's medication, since (unlike in a facility) compliance is a major issue. If you have not already done so, it would be helpful to know under what circumstances your patient wants to be transferred to the hospital. Finally, contact with this man's family and an understanding with him about who is to make decisions for him about health care in the event that he is incapable of doing so himself will be important and may require flexibility on your part.

13.1

The yearly history and physical examination, formerly considered a marker for good medical care, is often perfunctory and is rarely productive. Yearly reevaluation of mental status, medications, activities of daily living independence, list of medical problems, and advance directives is probably better. The necessary frequency of routine visits in stable nursing home patients is controversial. Most experienced physicians and administrators would agree that a visit every two weeks is unnecessary and wastefully expensive. Once a year is probably too infrequent, even for the least complex patient. Every 3 to 6 months may be a reasonable compromise. Tuberculosis screening makes a preadmission chest x-ray a reasonable demand. Medical availability seems to us necessary, and adequate nursing home care is not possible without a full set of records in the facility.

Please return to page 106 for further clinical exercises.

13.2

Advance directives are an essential part of nursing home care. The four categories outlined on the form are fairly typical of directives in many facilities. There seem to us to be two problems with this form. First, it is not clear whether the patient herself is to be consulted on which advance directive is chosen. Second, we believe that the delegation of a substituted decision-maker to assist with decision-making not covered by these somewhat artificial four categories is very important. The substituted decision-maker, of course, would be used only if the patient herself was unable to make a particular decision. Please carry on with the exercises on page 106.

13.3

This is a classic example of the scheduling and structural problems that exist between the nursing home and primary care physician. We believe that it is reasonable, in this situation, to request that the nurse who contacts you have seen the patient herself, that there be some physical as well as historical information, and that the nurse have a professional opinion about the urgency of the situation. Visiting this patient after the end of your office hours is probably sufficient, but unless the nurse has seen the patient and can provide vital information, you are unable to make the judgment. Obviously, there is pressure for care of other people both on the nurse and yourself in this circumstance. Patience is a virtue.

Carry on with Chapter 14.

14.1

Pentazocine is not known to be an effective narcotic in cancer pain management. Although individuals may vary, we favor and recommend the use of codeine, oxycodone, morphine, or hydromorphone. Read over the section on pain control in the summary of Chapter 14 (page 191) before continuing with this case on page 111.

14.2

Morphine is a more effective narcotic than pentazocine. Classically, sustained-release morphine is not given until a daily morphine requirement is established using normal-release medication. Often, however, this can be done by starting out with a low dose of sustained-release morphine and then adding further short-acting morphine for (breakthrough) pain. This would be our favorite drug treatment option here, but there is, strictly speaking, no pain diagnosis. Review the section on pain management in the summary of Chapter 14, page 191, and then turn to page 111 to continue with this case.

14.3

This is the most effective medication choice for this patient. It is important, however, to establish a pain diagnosis before undertaking treatment. Physical examination is both reassuring (and on occasion) revealing. Review the section on pain management in the summary of Chapter 14, page 191, and then turn to page 111 to continue with this case.

14.4

Although drug treatment is going to be critical here, physical examination is, we agree, a reasonable first step. Turn back to page 111 for the rest of this case.

14.5

Antihistamines are most effective for nausea originating from the labyrinth. Dimenhydrinate has a sedating effect that may be beneficial, but in general it would not be our first choice in this situation, where stomach emptying is likely to be the cause of the problem. Reread the options for nausea control in the summary of Chapter 14, page 192, before proceeding with Chapter 15.

14.6

This drug and other phenothiazines are beneficial when nausea originates from the chemoreceptor trigger zone. This might be effective in this situation, and it would be our second-choice medication. Prokinetic drugs that encourage gastric emptying are a bit more likely to be effective. Reread the list of options in the summary of Chapter 14 on page 192 before proceeding with Chapter 15.

14.7

Prokinetic drugs such as metoclopramide are probably the most effective first choice in this situation. Although metoclopreamide can have central nervous system (CNS) side effects, it is less expensive than domperidone and cisapride and so should, in our opinion, be tried first. Carry on with Chapter 15.

14.8

This patient is becoming dehydrated. Symptomatic drug treatment of her nausea is reasonable, and we would use metoclopramide first. Carry on with Chapter 15.

Part II   Notes on Geriatrics

Chapter 1—Aging and Frailty

I. Aging
  A. Demographics—The coming tide
    1. Life expectancy has increased
    2. The population pyramid is squaring
    3. Huge proportional increase in over-85s

  B. Who are the elderly?
    1. Mostly women (48% at age 65; 54% at 70; 71% at 85; 78% at 100)
    2. Many alone
    3. Increasingly well educated
    4. Most not wealthy
    5. More disabled with age (5% in facility at 65; 22% at 85)
    6. Remember the atypical

  C. Why do we age? (nobody knows, but . . .)
    1. Genetic theories (biological clock runs out, cell doublings limited, evolutionary function fulfilled)
    2. Stochastic (means according to probability)
      • Errors and mutations
      • Toxins (free radicals, radiation, metabolic products)
      • Autoimmunity
    3. Naturally selected, there would be no mechanism for an organism to evolve characteristics to extend its life beyond the mean age at which it would die from external (predatory, climatic) causes. We're trapped by our wild ancestors' lifespans.

D. Changes of normal aging
  1. The Rule of "3s": one third disuse, one third disease, one third normal aging
  2. A few specific generalities
     • Sleep is interrupted
     • Sexuality diminishes
     • Organ system function declines
     • All changes are marked by wide variability: the principle of heterogeneity

E. Psychosocial aging
  1. "Success" may be a balance between staying in training and gracefully disengaging
  2. Personalities are stable after age 30: we become more like ourselves (more still with aging, for better or worse)

F. Successful aging
  Can lifestyle modification minimize the collapse of organ function that leads to frailty? Consider the success to date of prevention of heart disease, stroke, osteoporosis, cancer, and infectious disease.

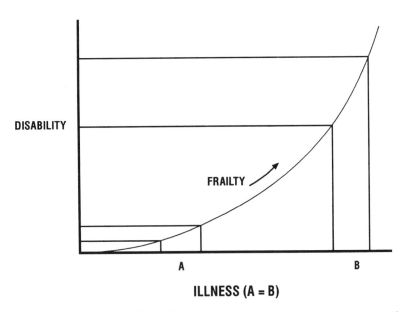

FIGURE 1.1. Frailty: The slippery slope (diagram courtesy David Brook, of Victoria, BC).

II. Frailty
   A. Defines our focus population (for research, care program planning, and payment)

   B. Frailty definitions
      1. The Brook graph and its slippery slope (Figure 1.1, page 150)
      2. Functional dependence
      3. Impaired but not too impaired: those we can probably help
      4. The dynamic model: resources on one side, millstones on the other; if the balance is tippy we can still make a difference

   C. Consequences of frailty
      1. The need for care: disabilities require support
      2. Our health care focus changes: function and quality of life come first
      3. Traditional evaluation doesn't work any more. Enter comprehensive geriatric assessment (see Chapter 2)

Chapter 2—Comprehensive Geriatric Assessment

I. Introduction
    A. This is the tool for our target population: the frail elderly; when you identify frailty, turn on comprehensive geriatric assessment (CGA)

    B. Where? Anywhere: office, nursing home, acute care, patient's home, geriatric unit; the principles remain the same

    C. Why so comprehensive?
        1. Problems are complex and tend not to go away.
        2. Maintaining independence and support is a continuing juggling act.
        3. Multiple disciplines always involved.

II. The Four Basic Steps (Figure 2.1)
    A. Baseline

    B. Excellent professional assessment

    C. Formulation

    D. Intervention
        1. The process proceeds around clockwise.
        2. It continues indefinitely.
        3. Case manager and case conference are essential.

III. Baseline
    A. Activities of daily living and instrumental activities of daily living (ADL/IADL)
        1. The central measurement of geriatrics
        2. Advancing frailty is measured by sequential failure of these functions

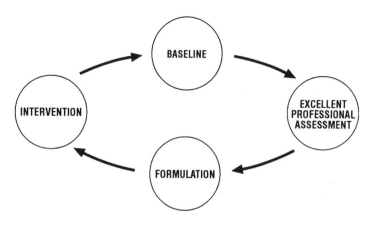

FIGURE 2.1. Four basic steps of comprehensive geriatric assessment.

    3. Remember the mnemonics:
       Dressing
       Eating
       Ambulating
       Toiletting
       Hygiene

       Shopping
       Housework
       Accounting (banking)
       Food preparation (cooking)
       Transport
    4. May be reported or performed (tested)
    5. Must be supported where failed

B. Cognition
    1. Higher mental, cortical, or brain function; includes memory, orientation, calculation, insight, abstraction, and judgment
    2. Relatively easy to measure (but beware some pitfalls): Folstein MMSE (Figure 2.2, p. 154), short portable mental status questionnaire, 3MS, neuropsych testing
    3. Beware delirium!

C. Social supports
    1. May require collateral history and confirmation by visit.

FOLSTEIN
MINI MENTAL STATUS EXAM

Date: _____   Examiner: _____

Score   ORIENTATION

(   )   What is the (year) (season) (month) (date) (day)   (5 pts)

(   )   Where are we? (country) (province) (city)   (5 pts)
                    (hospital) (floor)

              REGISTRATION

(   )   Name 3 objects: One second to say each. Then   (3 pts)
                    ask the patient to repeat all
                    three after you have said them.
                    One point for each correct.
                    Then repeat them until he
                    learns them. Count trials and
                    record _____

              ATTENTION AND CALCULATIONS

(   )   Serial 7s. One point for each correct answer. Stop
              at 5 answers. *Or* spell "world" backwards.
              (No. correct = letters before first mistake)   (5 pts)

              RECALL

(   )   Ask for the objects above. One point for each cor-   (3 pts)
              rect.

    (21)

              LANGUAGE TESTS
(   )   Name: pencil, watch   (2 pts)
(   )   Repeat: no ifs, ands, or buts   (1 pt)
(   )   Follow a three-stage command:
              "Take the paper in your right hand, fold it in half,   (3 pts)
              and put it on the floor."

(   )   Read and obey the following:
(   )   Close your eyes.   (1 pt)
              Write a sentence spontaneously below.   (1 pt)

(   )   Copy design below.   (1 pt)
    (9)

_____ Total (30 pts)

(   )

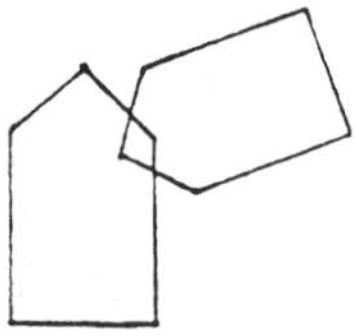

FIGURE 2.2. The Folstein Mini-Mental Status Examination.

    2. Should correspond to ADL/IADL deficiencies.
    3. The caregiver is the key to success.
    4. Plan ahead; try to arrange "safety net."

IV. Excellent Professional Assessment
    A. The *biggest* evaluation in health care
      1. Much more detail than the tedious primary care once-over
      2. More comprehensive than the focused specialist's "scope"

    B. History ABCs (vital information)
      1. ADL/IADL
      2. Brain failure (time course; possible causes)
      3. Collateral history (family, professionals)
      4. Drugs and alcohol (include compliance and watch for misinformation)
      5. Emotional, behavioral, psychological problems (including past psychiatric history)
      6. Falls and mobility failure
      7. Guardianship, caregiver and placement (if incapable, what is in place?)
      8. Hazards: fire, driving, abuse
      9. Incontinence

    C. Physical evaluation ABCs (measuring performance)
      1. Ambulation (balance and gait assessment)
      2. BP changes (with position)
      3. CNS and MSK (the two forgotten systems: vital in the elderly)
      4. Cognition (a quantitative evaluation)
      5. Competence (of person and finances: able to make decisions?)
      6. Drug-taking and alcohol evidence (find and count the pills and the bottles)
      7. Environment (evaluate the safety hazards and challenges)
      8. Function (ADL and IADL performance)

V.   Formulation
    A. The comprehensive problem list

1. After *all* the information is in, sit down and make a list (usually a very long list).
2. Include everything of possible relevance; this is the summary of all health data.

B. The remediable problem list
1. Evaluate and list the problems you think you might be able to fix.
2. This forms the basis for intervention.

VI. Intervention
A. Bring your best guesses about remediability to the multidisciplinary conference (or some approximation of it).
B. Set up a well-documented specific plan: what first, who does it, when evaluated?
C. Conduct careful intervention.

VII. Return to Baseline—Reevaluate Function After Each Intervention

VIII. The Circle Continues.

Chapter 3—Prescribing in the Elderly

I. Introduction
   A. Difficulty with drugs in elderly occurs for three un-avoidable reasons:
      1. Multiple pathology leads to multiple prescribing (the elderly, sicker on the average than young people, tend to be on more meds).
      2. Heterogeneity: elderly differ from one another in important determinants of drug consequences (eg, renal function, body water, receptor affinity).
      3. Compliance: variable and unpredictable

   B. Result: Unpredictability
      When you give medication to an elderly person you *don't know* what the result will be.

   C. Sometimes prescribing is simply inappropriate ("polypharmacy") because
      1. Treating symptoms: no diagnosis
      2. Wrong drug for condition or for elderly
      3. Right drug, wrong dose
      4. Too many drugs

II. The Ten Rules for Prescribing in the Elderly (or, how to keep polypharmacy down to a dull roar)
      1. Don't—If you can use no meds or one med (instead of three), do so.
      2. Start low—Lower doses, often 1/4 usual adult starting dose, are safer.
      3. Go slow—Titrate dosage upward in small increments; allow extra time for steady state.
      4. Never start treatment without clear end points in mind—Outcome of a drug prescription may be *ben-*

efit, *ADR* (adverse drug reaction), *both*, or *neither*; know how to measure which occurs.

5. Always return to measure the outcome—The most common error is not to do this; once there, see what outcome you have, take the rational next step, and arrange to return again.

6. Review the medication at every visit—Drug list in the facility, pill bottle at home, plastic bag in the office; never see anyone without knowing what they're taking, and explain to them or family the reason, dose, expected response.

7. Risk reducing drugs regularly—Unnecessary medications accumulate (other doctors, wrong diagnoses, temporary conditions); pick a potentially toxic drug, reduce it in small slow increments, return to measure outcome, and take the rational next step; this is the reverse of starting medication and titrating.

8. One thing at a time—If two drugs are started while one is being reduced, overall benefit may have several causes.

9. Ensure compliance—You can't reasonably do anything with medication until you know directions are followed. Blister pack, explain, supervise, simplify, and then evaluate compliance. Prescribing without it is gas on a fire.

10. Keep it simple—The fewer the drugs, the less frequently, the better for the patient, nursing, and the doctor.

III. Other Prescribing Principles
   A. Titrate to function (ADL), the final common pathway, best indicator of success or trouble, and most important outcome to patient.
   B. Never underestimate compliance traps: sudden changes in compliance may cause problems from rebound illness or adverse drug reaction.
   C. Learn and practice the treatment of high-risk, high-yield conditions; these include depression, Parkinson's disease, agitation, and musculoskeletal pain.

D. Nobody is ever stable; frail elderly people require routine surveillance even when no treatment is changing; schedule your return visits according to risk.

E. Somebody is paying the bill; use the least expensive safe, effective compound.

Chapter 4—Mobility Failure

I. Introduction
   A. Mobility failure is falling, unsteadiness, or immobility; it is a geriatric giant.
   B. Mobility is as necessary for function (ADL) as cognition and is harder to measure.
   C. Everyone sees gait and balance differently: ask a neurologist, a physiotherapist, a psychiatric social worker, and a facility nurse.
   D. This big topic takes lots of time, attention to detail, common sense, and a persistent multidisciplinary approach.

II. Normal Mobility
   A. Consists of balance, walking, and response to challenges.
   B. Many functions and systems involved and necessary: vision, neck mechanoreceptors, labyrinthine balance, proprioception/cerebellar coordination, cerebral cortex, motor system, bones/muscles/joints, affect/attitude, environment and support.
   C. All of these 'normally' age: many decondition, many get remediably sick.

III. The Specific Mobility Evaluation
   A. Add gait and balance assessment to your repertoire.
   B. "Get up and go" test (may be timed)
      1. From sitting in hard chair with no arms: stand momentarily, walk 3 meters toward wall, turn, return, sit.
      2. Watch for two things:
         a. Safety
         b. What is the diagnosis?

C. Watching someone walk (less formal) or standard mobility instruments (more formal): same process, same issues

IV. Finding Remediable Mobility Failure Causes
   A. There are a thousand causes; most of them you can't fix.

   B. Follow our mnemonic for "high yield" causes that you can.

   C. The mobility failure history (CATASTROPHE):
      Caregiver and housing
      Alcohol
      Treatment (drugs)
      Affect
      Syncope
      Teetering (dizziness)
      Recent illness
      Ocular problems
      Pain with mobility
      Hearing
      Environmental hazards

   D. The mobility failure physical evaluation (I HATE FALLING):
      Inflammation of joints

      Hypotension (orthostatic)
      Auditory and visual test
      Tremor (or other findings) of parkinsonism
      Equilibrium (balance) testing

      Foot problems
      Arrhythmia, heart block, valve disease
      Leg length discrepancy
      Lack of conditioning
      Illness (signs of)
      Nutrition poor
      Gait disturbance

   E. Don't forget the home visit (CHAT):
      Caregiver and housing
      Hazards

       Alcohol
       Taking medication properly?

V. Mobility Failure Treatment
    A. Tackle the problem with full comprehensive geriatric assessment (see Chapter 2)

    B. Identify and treat remediable causes

    C. Mobility intervention checklist:
       Environmental hazards
       Home supports
       Socialization and encouragement
       Modify medication*
       Balance training*
       Modify restraints
       Involve family
       Facility and homemaker
       Followup

---

* Shown to be most likely to make a difference in controlled trial

Chapter 5—Incontinence

I.   Introduction
   A. A common and very unpleasant symptom, often hidden due to embarrassment
   B. Hard on caregivers, no matter how dedicated
   C. A geriatric giant: often reversible when acute
   D. Is it incontinence? Ask the patient or caregiver: people's standards vary.

II. Practical Bladder Physiology (Figure 5.1)

III. Clinical Classification (The frailer the patient, the more blurred and less useful these categories)
   A. Stress incontinence: small volume of urine escapes when laughing or coughing increases abdominal pressure; incompetence of the internal sphincter
   B. Urge incontinence: unable to hold water soon after feeling the urge to void; often unstable bladder
   C. Overflow incontinence: continuous dribbling due to urine escaping in an obstructed or atonic bladder

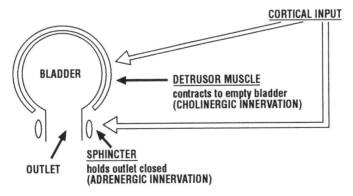

FIGURE 5.1. Functioning of the bladder.

IV. Algorithm for Incontinence Evaluation (Figure 5.2)

V. Specific Incontinence Treatment
   A. Predisposing causes, infection, and impaction: treat as indicated to remedy the problem

   B. Outlet obstruction
      1. Males—Finasteride may help: if likely benign, trial of therapy probably worthwhile; try alpha-blockers (prazosin, others); urology referral for persisting obstruction unless advanced disability (catheter)
      2. Female—If previously cystoscoped and known benign stricture, consider office or facility dilatation; otherwise refer for relief of obstruction.

   C. Atrophic urethritis—Topical or oral estrogen unless contraindicated

   D. Pure stress incontinence
      1. Kegel exercises
      2. Drugs (estrogen, pseudoephedrine, propranolol, alpha-agonists) usually not practical
      3. Surgery (suprapubic bladder suspension, more elaborate procedure)

   E. Atonic bladder—bethanachol

   F. Unstable bladder (detrusor instability or bladder dyssynergy)
      1. Drugs (oxybutinin, propantheline, dicyclomine, flavoxate, nifedipine, imipramine)
      2. Bladder retraining (timed voiding, biofeedback)

   G. DHIC (detrussor hyperactivity impaired contractility)
      1. Seeming contradiction in terms, rarely a rewarding practical diagnosis
      2. Try imipramine

   H. Mixed incontinence
      1. Try to sort out causes and treat with least invasive and toxic option
      2. Always try bladder training

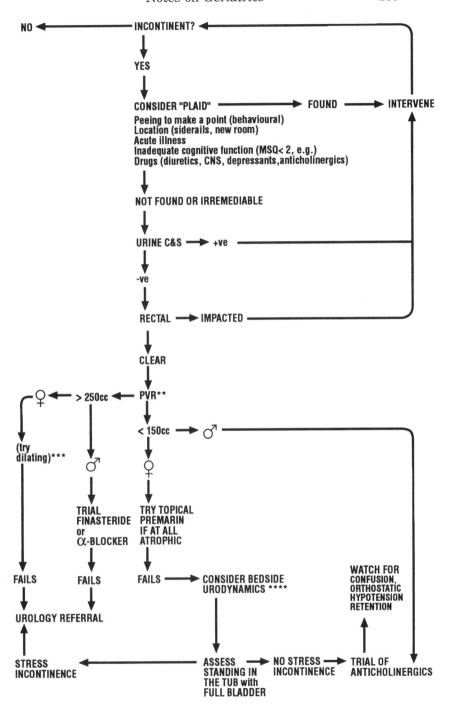

FIGURE 5.2. Incontinence evaluation.

I.   The bottom line—containment systems
     Pad and diapers nearly always superior to catheter and
     condom.

VI. Fecal Incontinence—See Chapter 9

Chapter 6—Cognitive Impairment

I. Introduction
    A. The aging brain is a sensitive organ; any disturbance can cause its temporary failure

    B. The two great brain syndromes
        1. Delirium: insult to aging brain causes acute failure
        2. Dementia: specific illness or injury causes permanent damage
        (don't forget acute-on-chronic: both at once)

    C. Real reversible cognitive impairment is probably rare (even in delirium), but its impact can be minimized by good medical and social care

II. Confusion Triage (Figure 6.1)

III. Delirium
    A. DSM-IV criteria
        1. Change of consciousness and loss of attention
        2. Cognitive change or perceptual disturbance
        3. Time course short and fluctuating
        4. Various causes are specified.

    B. The urgency of delirium
        1. Causes may be dangerous and treatable.
        2. Recent literature suggests delirium often *not* reversible.

    C. Common causes (CAMP squared)
        CHF, CNS (subdural, stroke)
        Alcohol, acute abdomen
        Metabolic (blood test accessible), medication
        Pyrexial (infection), psychological

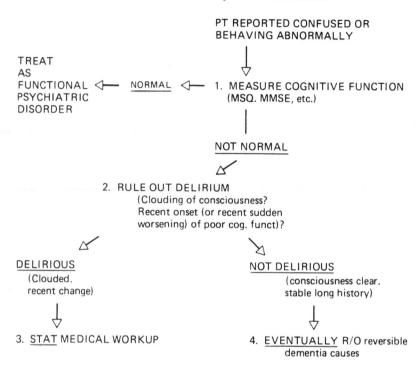

FIGURE 6.1. Confusion triage.

    D. Symptomatic treatment
        1. Reassurance and nonthreatening environment
        2. Benzodiazepines or careful neuroleptics

IV. Dementia
    A. DMS-IV criteria
        1. Cognitive deficit
           a. Memory impairment
           b. One or more of aphasia, apraxia, agnosia, decreased executive function
           c. Significant decrease in social function
           d. Criteria specific to various dementia causes

    B. Causes or syndromes
        1. Alzheimer's disease
        2. Vascular (formerly multiple infarct)
        3. Trauma
        4. Alcohol ("substance induced persisting")

5. Degenerative diseases (Parkinson's, Pick's, Huntington's)
6. Mixed
7. Frontal or frontoparietal syndromes

C. So-called reversible causes
1. The famous mneumonic DEMENTIA does not really identify many reversible causes, but it is useful in going over the possibilities and some co-morbidity:
>Drugs
>Emotional
>Metabolic
>Eyes/ears
>Nutritional/neurological
>Tumors and trauma
>Infection
>Atherosclerosis, alcohol, anemia
2. Be aware of subdural hematoma, normal pressure hydrocephalus, and toxic/metabolic states

D. Treatment
1. Drugs: many have claimed to improve Alzheimer's disease (most recently tacrine); any benefit usually early stages and temporary
2. Good comprehensive evaluation may identify contributing factors and partial remediability
3. Caregiver support: factor most strongly related to avoiding institutionalization
4. Management of psychological symptoms without drug toxicity challenging and essential

V. Cognitive Measurement for Nonneuropsychologists
A. Folstein MMSE (Figure 2.2, page 154); Short Portable Mental Status Questionnaire
1. Numerical-score cognitive measurement instruments
2. Limitations are lack of sensitivity and specificity.
3. Strengths are reproducibility, and superiority to "orientation ×3."

B. Tests for delirium measure attention: serial subtraction, digit span

Chapter 7—Depression

I. Introduction
   A. Very common in the elderly, especially males; suicide common, too

   B. Confusing to diagnose and treat because:
      1. Clouded by physical illness and medication
      2. Complex relationship with cognitive impairment
      3. Confused with normal aging: slowing down, sleep and dietary changes, mistaken low expectation for enjoying life: "he's old, he should be depressed about it."

   C. Criteria for mood disorders not reliable in elderly; careful trial of treatment may be necessary.

II. Terminology à la DSM-IV
   A. Major depressive episode (MDE): this is two weeks of five of the famous criteria, known by many mnemonics:
      Anhedonia
      Dysphoria
      Weight or appetite change
      Sleep disturbance
      Psychomotor rate change
      Fatigue or loss of energy
      Guilt or worthlessness
      Poor concentration or indecisiveness
      Suicide attempt, ideation, or thoughts of death

   B. Major depressive disorder: MDE not due to other illness, and without mania (single episode or recurrent)

C. Consider also
  1. Dysthymia—two-year history of depressed mood without MDE
  2. Simple bereavement or adjustment disorder (depressed mood)—unhappiness is clearly associated with major psychosocial stressor
  3. Dementia—cognitive impairment clearly present and dominates the clinical picture
  4. Non-DSM: morbid grief

III. Secondary Depression
  A. Mood disorder due to a medical condition or substance should be ruled out: may respond to treating underlying condition; difficult to treat as depression

  B. Drugs: theoretically, any drug can contribute, but consider especially:
    1. Old-fashioned antihypertensives
    2. Narcotic analgesics
    3. NSAIDs
    4. L-dopa
    5. Sedatives
    6. Steroids
    7. Alcohol

  C. Chronic disorders: any major medical condition, but especially those associated with pain

IV. Atypical Presentation of Depression
  A. The elderly *may* have full-blown classic depressive features

  B. More likely, their depression is partly hidden or goes unrecognized unless you consider the following presentations:
    1. Somatization—numerous complaints, especially without much physical basis
    2. Alcohol—new onset of heavy drinking in an elderly person
    3. Agitation—especially in cognitively impaired people

4. Withdrawal—social isolation
5. Pain—complaints of pain with nonorganic features may be "depression equivalent"
6. Geriatric failure to thrive—decreased ADL ability
7. Self-neglect

V. Depression and Cognition
   A. Elderly people may be depressed, cognitively impaired or both
   B. If depressed, the mood will respond to treatment
   C. If poor cognitive performance is secondary to depression, cognitive performance will improve; likelier, only the mood will respond

VI. Treatment of Depression
   A. Psychotherapy *is* successful sometimes, but rarely as the only modality

   B. Biological treatment often requires a careful trial according to the principles of drug therapy in Chapter 3

   C. Drugs of choice:
      1. SSRIs
         a. Now the first choice antidepressants in the elderly outpatient (they *do* cause side effects but less serious ones than TCAs), *except* some experts use TCAs first for severe depression
         b. Initial weight loss and agitation are the usual problems
         c. Doses should be low, monitoring careful, and trial periods lengthy—up to six weeks.
         d. If one drug doesn't work, another may.
         e. Fluvoxamine, sertraline, and paroxetine are superior to fluoxetine because of shorter half life and fewer interactions.
      2. Moclobemide—selective MAO inhibitor, effective in MDE and depression with Parkinson's; use adequate doses
      3. Tricyclic antidepressants—delirium, orthostatic hypotension, and urinary retention makes these

dangerous; use OK if previously successful without adverse drug reactions or in SSRI failure
4. Consider adding lithium (low blood level) or L-thyroxine to potentiate antidepressants.
5. Consider nortriptyline and SSRI in combination or venlafaxine, which may combine benefits of both.

D. Electroconvulsive Therapy
1. Good and effective treatment in elderly who don't tolerate or respond to drugs
2. May require maintenance treatment.

Chapter 8—Abuse, Alcohol, and Automobiles

I. Introduction
   A. Elderly people experience similar social problems to those seen in humans of all ages.
   B. Their response is influenced by aging: frailty, disability, and atypical presentation are usually important.

II. Elder abuse
   A. May be physical, emotional, sexual, nutritional, or financial
   B. May be active or passive (neglect).
   C. Profile of typical abused
      1. Female
      2. Dependent physically
      3. Controls finances
      4. Difficult-to-care-for problem
      5. Cognitively impaired, especially behaviorally difficult
   D. Profile of typical abuser
      1. Single caregiver; severe burden of care
      2. Financially dependent on elder who receives care
      3. Difficult or aggressive personality
      4. Substance abuser
   E. Look for injury (especially unusual ones), weight loss, failure to thrive, poor hygiene: all may appear to be simple consequences of aging.
   F. Under-reporting: fear of reprisal and abandonment
   G. Management: Assure safety, then provide assistance with caregiving, counselling and super-

vision; try to maintain the caregiving situation if possible.

III. Alcohol
   A. Sometimes on the bottom row in the "house of cards": frail elderly may depend on alcohol and collapse if it is removed.

   B. Diagnosis
      1. Presentation not typical: confusion, falls, incontinence, fail to thrive, withdrawal in hospital, suicide attempt
      2. Screen with CAGE questions:
         Cutting down fails
         Annoyance re habit
         Guilt
         Eye-openers
      3. Three types of elderly drinkers
         a. Late starters
         b. Life-long alcoholics who somehow survived
         c. Symptomatic (of depression or pain)
      4. Major problems with under-reporting and denial

   C. Treatment
      1. Abstinence often not a realistic goal; consequence can be collapsing frailty.
      2. Try to build rapport gradually, reassure that abrupt changes won't occur.
      3. Avoid confrontation.
      4. Try to tie unwanted symptoms to alcohol use
      5. Seek control of intake, relief of symptoms, and limitations of frailty.

IV. Driving
   A. Changes of aging decrease reaction time, cause visual and hearing impairment.

   B. Older drivers generally can be safe but must be cautious.

   C. Public safety must be weighed against unfairly imposing dependence (IADL disability).

D. Driving may be limited (highway, nighttime, rush-hour) as partial option

E. Common problems causing increased accident risk:
   1. Seizures (fairly absolute contraindication)
   2. Arrhythmia (only if symptomatic)
   3. Angina (only if unstable)
   4. Arthritis (only if impairs neck turning and extremity dexterity)
   5. Parkinsonism
   6. Diabetes (only if true risk of hypoglycemia)
   7. Alcohol
   8. Medications (sedatives, insulin, tricyclic antidepressants)
   9. Cognitive impairment (see following)
   10. Visual impairment

F. The cognitively impaired driver:
   1. Motor system and vision may be spared.
   2. Problems are with motor planning and organizing.
   3. Complex traffic situations may be dangerous.
   4. Folstein score less than 20: probably impaired; less than 16: definitely impaired
   5. If in doubt, test on road.
   6. If patient judgment poor or your sixth sense suggests trouble, err on the side of safety.

Chapter 9—Constipation, Fecal Incontinence, and Pressure Sores

I. Introduction
   A. This triad of recurring and chronic problems are the preoccupation of a lot of extended care work.
   B. Subject to certain exceptions (see following), there is little truly new under the sun in treating these problems.
   C. Consistency and persistence pay off, whichever "formula" you use; results come slowly but surely.

II. Constipation
   A. There is a wide range of normal: as long as bowel movement occurs eventually and without discomfort, it is probably "normal."

   B. Expectations are high, and belief in the need for daily bowel movements hard to shake.

   C. Clear the way by eliminating specific causes:
      1. Drugs (dehydrators, anticholinergics)
      2. Painful anorectal lesions
      3. (Rarely) impending or subacute obstruction

   D. Provide bowel normalcy promotors
      1. High fiber substantial-bulk diet (root vegetables, fruit laxative, prunes, bran, etc)
      2. Maintain hydration (especially in summer; remember diuretics).
      3. Encourage mobility (including bed mobility).

   E. Clean out and regularize (This regime is one of at least 100. If you have your own use it; if not, try this one.)
      1. Evacuate the colon in whatever way necessary (enemas, suppositories, and/or laxatives).

2. Establish regular bowel movements in whatever way necessary, every 2 to 4 days, depending on the patient's "natural" rhythm.
3. Start with a mild laxative in the evening and a suppository in the morning after breakfast, followed by toileting.
4. If this routine works, gradually reduce and stop the laxative, and then eventually eliminate the suppository; this can take months.
5. If it doesn't work, change the interval (2 to 4 days), use a stronger laxative, repeat the clean-out, consider evaluating the GI tract.

III. Fecal Incontinence
   A. Referred to as "oozing" in our facility, it's a least favorite among care staff

   B. Very immobilized and cognitively impaired patients may have formed bowel movements in bed, which is preferrable to the disruption and pain of toileting; this is *not* fecal incontinence.

   C. Consider the mnemonic FECAL for causes:
      Fecal impaction
      Excess laxatives
      Cognitive or behavioural
      All diarrhea causes
      Local lesions

   D. If physical exam suggests impaction, clean out and regularize (see IIE, above).

   E. If persists once laxative regime established and enforced, rule out diarrhea causes and consider sigmoidoscopy to eliminate local tumors.

   F. Consider loperamide or codeine as appropriate and necessary.

IV. Pressure Sores
   A. Occur in the best-run facilities but more often in those others.

   B. Multiple etiology—consider them infarcts of skin and recall the following scheme for causes:

1. Systemic causes that impair oxygen and nutrition in the blood (anemia, hypoxia, poor nutrition)
2. Circulatory causes that impair blood delivery (atherosclerosis, diabetes, other vasculitis)
3. Local causes that compromise skin and impair healing (edema, infection, moisture)
4. The "bottom line": pressure and shearing force.

C. Shea classification

Grade I—erythema and warmth for 24 hrs
Grade II—into subcutaneous fat
Grade III—undermined beneath subcutaneous fat
Grade IV—to muscle and bone

D. We still recommend our old mnemonic POINTS:

Pressure and shearing (relieve and prevent them any way you can: turning, special beds, cushions, careful lifting).

Operate to debride necrotic tissue (this most-overlooked step requires a mini-operative approach by a physician).

Infection (we don't culture because results are always misleading; treat only delocalized cellulitis; the bugs are anerobes, staph, strep, and gram negatives).

Nursing care (we mean specific products for wounds; strong chemicals belong in the broom closet; try polymer and colloid products).

Treat general condition (anemia, malnutrition, hypoxia, congestive heart failure, etc; treat these if you see a realistic chance of improvement).

Surgery (flaps, grafts, etc are a last-ditch approach).

Chapter 10—Difficult Behavior

I. Introduction
   A. This is a heterogeneous grab-bag of problems with a final common pathway of the patient's being hard to care for because of behavior.

   B. Synonyms: agitation, sundowning, aggressiveness, wandering, etc

   C. Takes many forms: shouting, elopement, fighting with care, harming other residents, problems with food and elimination, etc.

   D. Can be one of your most difficult, persistent challenges.

II. Approaches to Diagnosis
   A. Bio-psycho-social-environmental cause classification:
      1. Biological (illness, medication, pain)
      2. Psychological (major psychiatric illness)
      3. Social (caregiver problems, conflict with other residents, misunderstanding, memories from past)
      4. Environmental (facility, physical annoyances)

   B. Medical-model differential diagnosis: "D is for agitation"
      1. Dolor—pain from any cause, often occult
      2. Drugs—SSRI, neuroleptic (akathisia), anticholinergic, *any* drug at all
      3. Delirium—see Chapter 6
      4. DSM-IV—Axis I psychiatric disorder: psychosis, agitated depression, mania (usually with psychiatric history)

5. Drainage—Fecal impaction and urinary retention; occult elimination problems in low-level patients
6. Disputes—caregiver stress issues: abuse, personality clash, cultural issues, misunderstanding, "sandwich generation" stresses
7. Dementia—just plain agitation in dementia; catastrophic outbursts and personality changes:
   a. Frontal lobe syndrome
   b. Organic personality disorder

Direct the history and physical examination to the above major causes.

C. Practical approach
   1. Response aggression: find and modify the external cause
   2. Spontaneous aggression: find and modify the internal cause

III. Approaches to Treatment
   A. The situation for caregivers is often difficult, even explosive: demonstrate a comprehensive effective approach at once.

   B. Make a tentative diagnosis and start a trial of treatment; hoofbeats are likely horse, not wildebeast.

   C. Identify and correct correctable causes, including undertaking drug therapy of specific illnesses

   D. Arrange for monitoring; you'll never know how you're doing unless someone objectively evaluates behavior.

   E. Begin behavior therapy:
      1. Educate caregivers.
      2. Correct social problems.
      3. Behavior modifiers need to be persistent; cognitively impaired people don't learn.

   F. Consider agitation symptom-management with drugs
      1. Benzodiazepines
         a. Often best for quick safe control

    b. Use simple, short-acting drugs (eg, alprazolam, temazepam)

    c. Try a basic dose, with "breakthrough prn"

    d. Danger: diazepam and lorazepam at low doses not safe

2. Neuroleptics

    a. Traditional agitation treatment; choose your side effects

    b. Extrapyramidal (Parkinsonism and akathisia) greatest with haloperidol, present with loxapine, least with thioridazine and risperidone

    c. Autonomic effects and sedation greatest with thioridazine, present with loxapine and risperidone, least with haloperidol.

    d. Loxapine often the best compromise; start low, go slow

    e. Risperidone: a complex drug; interactions and side effects may be bewildering (for MD); if in doubt, get geriatric psych help if it's available

3. Other options

    a. Antiepileptics (carbamazepine: rarely effective; valproate: more often works well; phenytoin: steer clear: too many ADRs)

    b. Narcotics (preneuroleptic psychosis treatment; sometimes the only option)

Chapter 11—The Team and Case Management

I. Introduction
    A. The frail elderly are complicated; nobody can handle their whole care alone
    B. The team may be very formal (academic evaluation unit with 40 employees), or very informal (a couple of professionals collaborating on a difficult patient).
    C. The team rolls on wheels of mutual respect, trust, and communication
    D. Case management means coordination of care; ideally, this eliminates wasteful redundancy without creating deficiencies in the service

II. Who's on the team
    A. Core members: nurse, physician, social worker—these functions are pretty well essential
    B. Next circle: physiotherapist, occupational therapist, pharmacist, nutritionist, others.
    C. Don't forget: home support worker, vehicle driver, family caregivers, and the patient (often called "client" in this setting).
    D. Anyone capable can case manage; all it takes is a genius for seeing the big picture, and computer-like attention to detail (characteristics of all geriatrics professionals . . .).

III. Flexibility of team roles
    A. The above team members define team functions (medical, direct care, social management)
    B. While sensitive to professional "turf" issues and realizing you can't replace a professional role, everyone can partially do others' roles in a pinch.
    C. Examples of role flexibility: nurse evaluates compliance, social worker assesses cognitive impairment,

physician evaluates mobility, physiotherapist assesses consequences of Parkinson's treatment during titration

IV. The basic team process (these steps are flexible, and may be formal or informal)
   A. Client identification and screening—who can you help; is this client one of them?
   B. Intake evaluation—more or less comprehensive geriatric assessment (see Chapter 2) by one or more core professionals
   C. Planning conference—everyone meets to discuss the problems, decide the course of evaluation and care, and assign responsibility
   D. Case manager designated
   E. Multidisciplinary assessment—relevant evaluation by professionals
   F. Progress conference
      a. Repeated reevaluations of problem list and how you're doing
      b. Reformulation of problems and plans
   G. Separation (if appropriate)—if setting is not primary care, a discharge plan and communication with receiving professionals

V. Team troubleshooting
   A. Conflict—usually leadership ambiguity or perceived professional role toe-treading; redefine who's doing what; don't overfunction
   B. Wrong clients, too many clients, too few clients
      a. Focus—stick to what you do best, and tackle the problems you can solve
      b. Pick the clients best suited to your program goals
   C. Personnel burn-out
      a. Build in time for education and professional development
      b. Try socializing

Chapter 12—Home Care and Caregiver Support

I. Introduction
   A. Types of home care
      1. Hospital replacement—home IV and early discharge
      2. Short- and long-term care at home—may be the frail elderly care venue of the future.
      3. Palliative care
      4. "Quick response"—short intense support at home to avoid admission from ER

   B. Why give care at home?
      1. Improved quality—some of what is futile, dangerous, expensive, and morbidity-promoting in hospital care is replaced with safer, more dignified, and custom-designed care.
      2. Most elderly clients prefer being at home and recover more effectively.
      3. Cost-saving—it all started here, but the benefits go beyond the dollar.
      4. Funding can shift from wasteful expensive institutions to anticipatory home management.

II. The Physician in Home Care
   A. New breed of geriatric generalist: the home care doctor
   B. You must be a team player; you *won't* be the case manager and someone else (a nurse!) may tell you what to do and when.
   C. Fee-for-service payments probably are not a survivable method of remuneration in this situation.
   D. Professional reward: an excellent and thorough job based on physical diagnosis, trial of therapy, me-

ticulous follow-up, and cooperation among professionals

E. The office shifts to the home, the car, the adult day center, the facility, and community health clinics.

F. As primary physician you can discourage unnecessary referrals: blow the whistle on subspecialist volleyball.

III. Tools of the Home Care Trade: How to Make It Work

A. Adult day center—respite, socialization, medical care, and other health services: bring home care patients in for economies of similar services

B. Anticipatory focus—you and the team know all the problems and the likely worst case scenarios and are ready to handle them.

C. Immediate response to crisis—the patient and caregiver are reassured, and their care is optimized by your "911-style" 24-hour response to calls for help.

D. A single medical record—the home care health team is the case manager, and all information is available in one place

E. Institutions are very special needs resources (planned or crisis respite, short convalescence); hospitals and nursing homes are no longer the default venues.

F. Least required service provider—health care workers do much monitoring, nurses follow chronic illness, general physician makes most medical and psychiatric diagnoses and decisions.

G. Conferencing—the whole team is made aware of the status, the plans, and any changes.

H. Compliance surveillance—the home-care elderly are pharmacological accidents waiting for a chance to happen: know your meds; use your pharmacist.

I. Caregiver and caregiver support—see following.

J. The right patient—wants home care; preferably illness and terminal care at home; not red lights, siren, and TV-series ER/ICU action.

K. Advance directives—plan for the long term, set goals with patient and families; don't forget delegation of a capable substituted decision-maker.

IV. Caregiver Support
   A. Patient outcomes are most closely tied to caregiver capability in literature.

   B. The services you provide are as much for the caregiver as for the patient.

   C. Education
      1. Groups: support and information
      2. Literature: books and information pamphlets
      3. One-on-one teaching of methods of care and what to expect
      4. Menu of services

   D. Counselling

   E. Respite—facility, overnight adult day care, or care provider in home: a rest is as good as a change

   F. Always deliver on your promise of prompt and thorough help and support—a worried caregiver is a "difficult" caregiver.

   G. Understand that many women as caregivers are employed at two jobs.

   F. Cut through or end-run bureaucratic tangles to get the kind of care that is really needed to its user

Chapter 13—Nursing Home Care

I. Introduction
   A. What is a nursing home?
      1. Names vary with venues
      2. Generally: light care (senior citizen's housing or personal care), intermediate care (nursing homes or ambulatory care), and heavy care (extended care or skilled nursing facility)
      3. A hybrid of home and hospital for dependent people requiring daily care; *not* acute care: staffing ratios don't permit intensive-style care.

   B. With movement toward more care in the community, facility patients have higher and higher impairment; tend to be cognitively impaired.

   C. Payment and administration issues vary; private versus public pay, private versus public administration.

   D. Multilevel facilities improve flexibility.

   E. Special units match wanderers and agitated with special staff and physical plant.

   F. Relocation stress needs your attention and sensitivity.

II. Characteristics of Nursing Home Care
   A. Generally, the population is the frailest and oldest, therefore care is most "geriatric": goals reflect this.
   B. More function-oriented, less focus on cure.
   C. More family and caregiver staff involvement, less patient capability; protection of autonomy requires flexible approach: remember incapacity isn't global.

    D. Major role for advance directives (degrees of intervention); may be misinterpreted and oversimplified.

    E. Emphasis on investigation and treatment in-home; less access to x-ray, hospital, invasive treatment, as a generality; *but* individual decisions essential.

    F. The medical job, done properly, is much *more* (not less) demanding of time and ability than that in the office.

III. The Doctor's Role

    A. "House doctor" versus staying with the former family doc: quality versus continuity of care

    B. Medical director: responsible for quality or responsible for filling the beds?

    C. MD teacher in the nursing home: medical students and residents; nursing home staff

    D. Types of medical visits:
      1. Initial evaluation: generate database, gather old records
      2. Specially called (emergency or nonurgent): availability is critical.
      3. Follow-up: every intervention creates a potential adverse outcome.
      4. Periodic evaluation: cognition, ADL, medication, advance directives, problem list; "routine" physical and blood work may not be effective; frequency controversial: depends on need.

IV. Documentation

    A. Must be legible, in the facility, portable, up to date.

    B. Contents:
      1. Problem list (ideally merge with other disciplines' plan)
      2. Progress notes (multidisciplinary or by discipline; legible and comprehensible to all caregivers)
      3. Medication list (justification for each drug)
      4. Record of cognition and ADL
      5. Advance directives
      6. Special reports (consults, x-rays, blood work)

V. Doctor/nurse cooperation
    A. If the hospital is a "doctors' shop", then nursing home is a "nurses' shop."
    B. Conflict of scheduling: doctor available early morning and before dinner; nurse available late shift (2 to 3 pm); dinnertime often impossible.
    C. Two short-fuse situations: doctor visits at mealtime, nurse telephones midafternoon
    D. Multidisciplinary conferences: the impossible rendezvous; these are essential and difficult to arrange.
    E. Collaboration is the answer: respect, trust, and communication; all are difficult and require an extra effort.

Chapter 14—Palliative Care

I. Introduction
   A. Palliative care meets the needs of very disabled or dying people when cure is no longer the primary goal.
   B. "To comfort always" should be a priority goal for all patients, not only those for whom we have exhausted frantic high-tech diagnostic and curative efforts.
   C. The best palliative healers control symptoms by combining technical capability and realistic reassurance; by showing you can help, you show you care.

II. Pain Control
   A. Pain is the most common symptom in cancer and other end-stage illness management.
   B. Total pain: treat the accompaniments and intensifiers of physical pain.
      1. Fear: death, loss of dignity, mutilation, and humiliation are terrifying prospects.
      2. Anger: treatment failures, bureaucracy and hassles; "Why me?"; a helpless bitter resentment can develop.
      3. Depression: every kind of loss, present and future, accumulate and threaten.
   C. Be objective: use a pain scale (0–5; 0–10).
   D. Analgesics: whatever the agent, use your pharmacokinetic knowledge to keep pain in control:
      1. Regular dosing plus breakthrough top-ups
      2. Keep the drug level above the pain threshold but below the level of sedation, except at night.
      3. Prevent constipation if using opioids.

E. Get familiar with effective narcotics (codeine, oxycodone, morphine, hydromorphone, others; *not* meperidine, pentazocine, propoxyphene), and learn to use them effectively in titration, maintenance, and step-up.

F. Use adjuvants for better control and lower narcotic dose:
   1. Nondrug (radiation, surgery, nerve blocks, acupuncture)
   2. Drug co-analgesics:
      a. NSAID (bone, soft tissue, hepatomegaly, arthritis)
      b. Corticosteroids (intracranial pressure, nerve compression, hypercalcemia, metastatic arthralgia)
      c. Benzodiazepines (anxiety, insomnia, muscle spasm)
      d. Neuroleptics (tenesmus, pain worse with anxiety)
      e. Antidepressants (dysaesthesia, neuralgia, depression)
      f. Anticonvulsants (intermittent neuralgia, dysaesthesia)
      g. Antiarrhythmics (mexiletene or flecainide for dysaesthesia)
      h. Antibiotics for cellulitis and infected ulcers
      i. Local anesthetic for mouth ulcers and skin breakdown
      j. Antispasmodics for muscle spasm
      k. Nitrous oxide for short intermittent painful episodes

III. Control of Other Symptoms
   A. Nausea and vomiting:
      1. Restrict oral intake and cut out intolerable foods.
      2. Phenothiazines (prochlorperazine, trifluoperazine), haloperidol
      3. Antihistamines (dimenhydrinate, others)
      4. GI kinetic (metoclopromide—watch CNS side effects—domperidone, cisapride)

5. Topical scopolamine
6. Steroids, benzodiazepines, THC

B. Bowel obstruction
   1. Partial relief is possible with certain drugs.
   2. Try atropine, hyoscine, belladonna/opium

C. Hiccup
   1. Paper bag rebreathing
   2. Chlorpromazine, diazepam, phenytoin
   3. Consider inducing gagging (gastric distention relief; vagal barrage)

D. Constipation
   1. Diet and fluids
   2. Irritants (sennosides) if moderate
   3. Suppository or enema if stool in rectum
   4. Oil retention enema, lactulose for resistant cases

E. Diarrhea
   1. Rule out fecal impaction
   2. Loperimide or opium

F. Cough
   1. Relieve tumor pressure with steroid or radiation
   2. Steam or salbutamol nebulizer
   3. Codeine, dextromethorphan

G. Dyspnea
   1. Standard medical differential diagnosis and care
   2. Morphine, neuroleptics, narcotics, atropine
   3. Oxygen is rarely symptomatically useful.
   4. Fans, airflow in room, and reassurance

Chapter 15—Ethical Issues

I. Euthanasia
   A. Permitting, assisting with, or causing someone's death in order to end a situation judged worse than death is controversial, and has been for millenia.

   B. Certain distinctions are possible
      1. Passive euthanasia
         a. Not providing clearly futile theoretically curative care is generally considered legitimate.
         b. Stopping initially possibly useful but subsequently clearly futile care: probably ethically no different from not starting treatment.
         c. Consensus and other professional opinions is comforting, morally and legally.
      2. Voluntary active euthanasia
         a. This is the most controversial type of "mercy killing."
         b. Defined as assisting in a suicide requested by a competent person.
         c. Arguments for: autonomy is paramount, acting and refraining are the same, forcing suffering is intolerable.
         d. Arguments against: traditional religious prohibition, ethical standards of profession, public sees physicians as executioners.
         e. Controversial and currently is illegal in most countries; a focus on extremely effective symptom control is a good healing compromise; exceptions may exist.
      3. Active nonvoluntary euthanasia: this is "mercy killing" of incompetent people whom we believe to have an intolerable experience of life; gener-

ally considered unethical and certainly every-
where illegal
4. Involuntary active euthanasia: killing against
someone's will (homicide)

II. Capability
A. Ability to perform mental tasks is required for
many human activities; making a will, managing
money, marrying, and consenting to treatment all
require ability to understand and decide

B. Capability laws are variable depending on circumstances and jurisdictions; when embarking on these
waters, know the law and keep a professional authority (lawyer) handy

C. Some principles for evaluating capability apply to
most situations:
1. Presume capability unless circumstances clearly
indicate otherwise
2. Always inform person being examined of reason
for examination.
3. Examining capability for a task establishes only
capability for *that* task (at that time), not for
others more or less complex
4. Evaluate cognition using recognized tests, evaluate affect and thought, make appropriate psychiatric diagnoses, and state severity.

D. Examine by questions the specific task at issue
(arithmetic and income/expenses etc. for finances;
best and worse outcomes for "yes" and "no" decisions
in consent to treatment).

E. Confirm statements of fact by reliable disinterested
collateral.

F. Make careful and clear notes; always assume you'll
be writing an important letter or talking alone in a
hushed courtroom.

G. When in doubt, get help, reevaluate, back off, and
refuse to conclude.

III. Care decisions for incompetent people

    A. If someone cannot decide on their care (cannot instruct you because they do not understand the issue), you as care provider have a problem.

    B. Follow guidelines for capability (see II above)

    C. The best solution is carefully prepared advance directives for care, including the name of a substituted decision-maker. It may of course be too late for that . . .

    D. Pursue a hierarchy:

        1. If incompetent, seek a previous decision ("living will" or equivalent) on *this* issue.

        2. If that is unavailable, seek a properly delegated substituted decision-maker and follow his or her instructions.

        3. If *that* is unavailable, make, in consultation with all involved and respecting known religious and ideological biases, a decision believed to be in the person's best interest.

Bibliography

Alexopoulos GS, Meyers BS, Young RC, et al. The course of geriatric depression with reversible dementia: a controlled study. *Am J Psychiatry.* 1993;150:1693–1699.

Allman RM, Laprade CA, Noel LB, et al. Air fluidized beds or conventional therapy for pressure sores—a randomized trial. *Ann Intern Med.* 1987;107:641.

Avorn J, Gurwitz JH. Drug use in the nursing home. *Ann Intern Med.* 1995;123(3):195–204.

Bayer AJ, Chadha JS, Farag RR, et al. Changing presentation of myocardial infarction with increasing old age. *J Am Geriatr Soc.* 1986;34:263.

Blazer DG, Federspiel CF, Ray WA, et al. The risk of anticholinergic toxicity in the elderly: a study of prescribing practices in two populations. *J Gerontol.* 1983;38:31.

Blazer DG. Is depression more frequent in late life? *Am J Geriatr Psychiatry.* 1994;2(3):193–199.

Boscia JA, Kobasa WD, Knight RA, et al. Therapy versus no therapy of bacteriuria in elderly ambulatory non-hospitalized women. *JAMA.* 1987;257:1067.

Boult C, Boult L, Murphy C, et al. A controlled trial of outpatient geriatric evaluation and management. *J Am Geriatr Soc.* 1994;42(5):465–470.

Brandeis GH, Ooi WL, Hossain M, et al. A longitudinal study of risk factors associated with formation of pressure ulcers in nursing homes. *J Am Geriatr Soc.* 1994;42(4):388–93.

Bressler R, Katz MD, eds. *Geriatric Pharmacology.* New York, NY: McGraw-Hill, Inc; 1993.

Buchsbaum DG, Buchanan RG, Welsh J, et al. Screening for drinking disorders in the elderly using the CAGE questionnaire. *J Am Geriatr Soc.* 1992;40(7):662–665.

Burke WJ, Rubin EH, Zorumski CF, Wetzel RD. The safety of ECT in geriatric psychiatry. *J Am Geriatr Soc.* 1987;35:526.

Clarfield AM: The reversible dementias: do they reverse? *Ann Intern Med.* 1988;109:476. Review.

Council on Scientific Affairs. American Medical Association. Physicians and family caregivers. A model for partnership. *JAMA.* 1993;269(10):1282–1284.

Dubeau CE, Resnick NM. Evaluation of the causes and severity of geriatric incontinence: a critical appraisal. *Urol Clin North Am.* 1991;18(2):243–256.

Duthie EH, Tresch DD. Use of CPR in the nursing home. *Nursing Home Medicine.* 1993;1(4):6–10.

Elbadawi A, Yalla, SV, Resnick NM. Structural basis of geriatric voiding dysfunction. I. Methods of a prospective utrastructural/ urodynamic study and an overview of the findings. *J. Urol.* 1993;150(5pt2):1650–1656.

Eslinger PJ, Damasio AR, Benton AL, et al. Neuropsychologic detection of abnormal mental decline in older persons. *JAMA.* 1985;253:670.

Ferrell BA, Keeler, E, Siu A, Ahn SH, Osterweil D. Cost-effectiveness of low-air-loss beds for treatment of pressure ulcers. *J Gerontol: Med Sci* (in press).

Finucane TF, Burtonb JR. Community-based long-term care. In: Hazzard WR, Bierman EL, Blass JP, et al, eds. *Principles of Geriatric Medicine and Gerontology.* New York, NY: McGraw-Hill, Inc. 1994:375–382.

Gerety MB, Cornell JE, Plichta DT, et al. Adverse events related to drugs and drug withdrawal in nursing home residents. *J Am Geriatr Soc.* 1993;41(12):1326–1332.

Gjorup T, Hendriksen C, Lund E, Stromgard E. Is growing old a disease? A study of the atttitudes of elderly people to physical symptoms. *J Chron Dis.* 1987;40:1095.

Groth-Juncker A, McCusker J. Where do elderly patients prefer to die? *J Am Geriatr Soc.* 1983;31:457.

Guam L, Ricciotti NA, Fair WR: Endoscopic bladder neck suspension for stress urinary incontinence. *J Urol.* 1984;132:1119.

Ham, R. *Primary Care Geriatrics.* Boston, Mass: John Wright. 1983.

High DM. Planning for decisional incapacity: a neglected area in ethics and aging. *J Am Geriatr Soc.* 1987;35:814.

Howell T, Watts DT. Behavioral complications of dementia: a clinical approach for the general internist. *J Gen Int Med.* 1990;5:431–437.

Jonsen A, Siegler M, Winslade W. *Clinical Ethics.* 3rd ed. New York, NY: Macmillan; 1992.

Judge JO, Whipple RH, Wolfson LI. Effects of resistive and balance exercises on isokinetic strength in older persons. *J Am Geriatr Soc.* 1994;42:937–946.

Kane RL, Williams CC, Williams TF, et al. Restraining restrains: changes in the standard of care. *Annu Rev Public Health.* 1993;14:545–584.

Kapp MB, compiler. Ethical Aspects of Health Care for the Elderly: An Annotated Bibliography. Westport, Conn: Greenwood Press; 1992.

Kroessler D, Fogel BS. Electroconvulsive therapy for major depression in the oldest old. *Am J Geriatr Psychiatry.* 1993;1(1):30–37.

Lewis MA, Kane RL, Cretin S, et al. The immediate and subsequent outcomes of nursing home care. *Am J Public Health.* 1985;75:758.

Magar RF. *Preparing Instructional Objectives.* 2nd ed. Belmont, Calif: John Wright; 1983.

Martin GR, Danner DB, Holbrook NJ. Aging—causes and defenses. *Annu Rev Med.* 1993;44:419–429.

Masur DM, Sliwinski M, Lipton RB, et al. Neuropsychological prediction of dementia and the absence of dementia in healthy elderly persons. *Neurology.* 1994;44(8):1427–1432.

Moos RH, Merten JR, Brennon PL. Patterns of diagnosis and treatment along late-middle-aged, and older substance abuse patients. *J Stud Alcohol.* 1993;54:479–487.

Nordenstam GR, Brandberg CA, Oden AS, et al. Bacteriuria and mortality in an elderly population. *N Engl J Med.* 1986;314:1152.

Ouslander JG. Geriatric urinary incontinence. *Dis Mon.* 1992;38(2):65–149.

Ouslander JG, Osterweil D. Physician evaluation and management of nursing home residents. *Ann Intern Med.* 1994;120(7):584–592.

Overstall PW, Hazell JWP, Johnson AL. Vertigo in the elderly. *Age Ageing.* 1981;10:105.

Pinchcofsky-Devin GD, Kaminski MV. Correlation of pressure sores and nutritional status. *J Am Geriatr Soc.* 1986;34:435.

Ray, WA, Griffin MR, et al. Psychotropic drug use and the risk of hip fracture. *N Engl J Med.* 1987;316:363.

Ray, WA, Taylor JA. Lichtenstein MJ et al. The nursing home behaviour problem scale. *J Gerontol.* 1992;47:9–16.

Risse SC, Barnes R. Pharmacologic treatment of agitation associated with dementia. *J Am Geriatr Soc.* 1986;34:368.

Robbins LJ, Boyko E, Lane J, et al. Binding the elderly: a prospective study of the use of mechanical restraints in an acute care hospital. *J Am Geriatr Soc.* 1987;35:290.

Roman GC, Tatemichi TK, Erkinjuntti T, et al. Vascular dementia: diagnostic criteria for research studies: report of the NINDS-AIREN International Workshop. *Neurology.* 1993;43(2):250–160.

Ross JL. *Long-Term Care: Current Issues and Future Directions.* Washington, DC: United States General Accounting Office. 1995; Publication no. GAO/HEHS-95-109.

Rubenstein LZ, Josephson KR, Robbins AS. Falls in the nursing home. *Ann Intern Med.* 1994;121:442–451.

Rubenstein LZ, Stuck AE, Siu AL, et al. Impacts of geriatric evaluation and management programs on defined outcomes: overview of the evidence. *J Am Geriatr Soc.* 1991;39(9pg2):8S–16S.

Sachs GA, Cassel CK, eds. Theme issue: Clinical Ethics. *Clin Geriatr Med.* 1994;(August):10.

Salzman C. *Geriatric Psychopharmacology.* 2nd ed. Baltimore, Md: Waverly Press; 1992.

Salzman C, Schneider L, Lebowitz B. Antidepressant treatment of very old patients. *Am J Geriatr Psychiatry.* 1993;1(1):21–29.

Sandman PO, Adolfsson R, Hallmans G, et al. Treatment of constipation with high-bran bread in long-term care of severely demented elderly patients. *J Am Geriatr Soc.* 1983;31:289.

Schiedermayer DL. The decision to forgo CPR in the elderly patient. *JAMA.* 1988;260:2096.

Stuck, AE, Siu AL, Wieland GD, et al. Comprehensive geriatric assessment: a meta-analysis of controlled trials. *Lancet.* 1993;342(8878):1032–1036.

Studenski S, Duncan PW, Chandler J, et al. Predicting falls: the role of mobility and nonphysical factors. *J Am Geriatr Soc.* 1994;42:297–302.

Sudarsky L, Ronthal M: Gait disorders among elderly patients: a survey study of 50 patients. *Arch Neurol.* 1983;40:740.

Teri L, Larson EG, Reifler BV: Behavioral disturbance in dementia of the Alzheimer's type. *J Am Geriatr Soc.* 1988;36:1.

Thibault JM, Maly RC. Recognition and treatment of substance abuse in the elderly. *Prim Care.* 1993;20(1):155–165.

Tinetti ME, Williams TF, Mayewski R. Fall risk index for elderly patients based on number of chronic disabilities. *Am J Med.* 1986;80:429.

Tinetti ME, Baker DI, McAvary G, et al. A multifactorial intervention to reduce the risk of falling among elderly people living in the community. *N Engl J Med.* 1994;331:821–827.

Vestal RE, Montamat SC, Nielson CP. Drugs in special patient groups: the elderly. In: Melmon KL, Morrelli HF, Hoffman BB, et al. eds. *Clinical Pharmacology—Basic Principles in Therapeutics.* 3rd ed. New York, NY: Macmillan; 1992:851–874.

Whitehead WE, Burgio KL, Engel BT: Biofeedback treatment of fecal incontinence in geriatric patients. *J Am Geriatr Soc.* 1985;33:320.

Index

A

Activities of daily living (ADL), 13. *See also* Comprehensive geriatric assessment
Adult day care center, 95–96
Advance directives, 116–117
Aging, 5–9, 149–151
  characteristics of, 5–6
  demographic factors, 5
  and disability, 6
  frail elderly, 8–9
  and lifestyle, 7–8
  notes on, 149–151
  psychosocial, 7
  theories of, 6
Agitation, and dementia, 50–51
Alcohol abuse, 63–64, 175
  and delirium, 48
  and dementia, 49
  and depression, 56, 57
  evaluation of, 63
  profile of elderly alcoholic, 63–64
  treatment of, 63
  withdrawal, 17, 63
Alpha-agonists, for incontinence, 43
Alprazolam, for difficult behavior, 82
Alzheimer's disease, 49–50
Ambulation, evaluation of, 17–18
Ambulatory care facilities, 100
Amnestic syndrome, 49
Angina, 25, 27
Antiarrhythmic drugs, for pain control, 109

Antibiotics, for pain control, 109
Anticholinergics
  for bowel obstruction, 110
  for incontinence, 43
Anticonvulsants, for pain control, 109
Antidepressants, for pain control, 109
Antihistamines, for nausea, 109
Antispasmodics, for pain control, 109
Assessment of elderly. *See* Comprehensive geriatric assessment (CGA)
Assisted suicide, 114
Atrophic urethritis, 43
Atropine, for shortness of breath, 110

B

Behavior. *See* Difficult behavior
Benign prostatic hypertrophy, and incontinence, 41, 43
Benzodiazepines
  for nausea, 110
  for pain control, 109
  side effects, 82
Beta blockers, 27
  for incontinence, 43
Bethanachol, for incontinence, 43
Biofeedback, 25
  for incontinence, 43
Bladder
  instability, 43
  normal functioning of, 39–40
  See also Incontinence

Bladder dyssynergy, 43
Blood pressure, evaluation of, 18
Brain failure, meaning of, 16

C

Calcium channel antagonists, 27
Capability of patient, 115–116
    evaluation of capability, 115–116
Carbamazepine, for difficult
    behavior, 83
Caregivers, support of, 98–99
Catheterization
    incontinence evaluation, 41
    incontinence treatment, 43
Central nervous system,
    evaluation of, 18
Central nervous system disease,
    and delirium, 48
Chlordiazepoxide, 82
Chlorpromazine, for hiccup, 110
Cisapride, for nausea, 109
Co-analgesia, for pain control,
    109
Codeine
    for cough, 110
    for pain control, 108
Cognitive assessment, 13–15, 18,
    46–48
    Folstein Mini Mental Status
        Exam, 14, 47, 51
    Short Portable Mental Status
        Questionnaire, 15, 47, 51
Cognitive impairment, 46–51,
    166–169
    confusion triage, 46–48
    delirium, 46, 48–49
    dementia, 46, 49–51
    and depression, 57–58
    notes on, 166–169
    and nursing home care, 100–
        101, 102
Collateral history, 16–17
Competence, evaluation of, 18
Compliance, medication-taking,
    27, 28
Comprehensive geriatric
    assessment (CGA), 11–20,
    152–155

activities of daily living,
    measurement of, 13
baseline information, 12–13
cognitive assessment, 13–15
history of patient, 16–17
instrumental activities of daily
    living, measurement of, 13
notes on, 152–155
physical evaluation, 17–19
remediable problem list, 19
and social supports, 15–16
team effort in, 11–12, 91–92
Congestive heart failure, 25, 27,
    28
    and delirium, 48
Constipation, 70–73, 177–178
    causes of, 71
    and fecal impaction, 71–72, 110
    and medication, 71
    treatment of, 71–72, 110
Corticosteroids
    for nausea, 110
    for pain control, 109
Cough, treatment of, 110

D

Decision making
    and nursing home care, 101–
        102
    substitute decision making,
        116
Delirium, 48–49
    causes of, 48–49
    and difficult behavior, 80
    DSM-IV criteria, 48
    evaluation of, 51
    meaning of, 46
Dementia, 28, 49–51
    causes of, 49–50
    and difficult behavior, 80
    DSM-IV criteria, 49
    evaluation of, 51
    meaning of, 46
    mixed dementia, 50
    reversible causes of, 50
    treatment approaches, 50
Depression, 27, 28, 36, 54–59,
    170–173
    atypical presentation of, 57

and cognitive impairment, 57–58
and dementia, 50–51
depressed mood, 55
DSM-IV criteria, 55–56
major depressive disorder, 55
major depressive episode, 55
morbid grief, 56
notes on, 170–173
secondary depression, 56–57
treatment of, 58–59
Desipramine, for depression, 58–59
Detrusor instability, 43
Dextromethorphan, for cough, 110
Diapers, for incontinence, 44
Diarrhea, treatment of, 110
Diazepam, 82
for hiccup, 110
Difficult behavior, 78–85, 180–182
causes of, 79–80
drug therapy for, 82–83
management of, 81–83
notes on, 180–182
types of behaviors, 78
Digoxin, 25
Diltiazem, 25
Documentation
capability evaluations, 116
nursing home, 104–105
Domperidone, for nausea, 109
Dopamine antagonists, for difficult behavior, 82
Driving by elderly, 64–66, 175–176
health problems interfering with, 65–66

E
Elder abuse, 61–63, 174–175
Elderly, assessment of, 11–20
Electroconvulsive therapy (ECT), for depression, 59
Environment, evaluation of, 18
Estrogens, for incontinence, 43
Ethical issues, 114–117, 194–196
advance directives, 116–117
capability, 115–116
euthanasia, 113–114
Euthanasia, 113–114
assisted suicide, 114
mercy killing, 114
Extended care facilities, 100

F
Falls. *See* Mobility failure
Family, and collateral history, 16–17
Fecal impaction, 71–72, 110
Fecal incontinence, 73, 178
Fever, and delirium, 48
Finasteride, for incontinence, 41, 43, 162
Flavoxate, for incontinence, 43
Fluoxetine
for depression, 58
and difficult behavior, 80
Flurazepam, 82
Fluvoxamine, for depression, 58
Folstein Mini Mental Status Exam, 14, 47, 49, 51, 66
Frail elderly, 8–9, 150, 151
changeability of, 20
characteristics of, 8–9, 149
support services for, 9
Frontoparietal dementias, 50

G
Geriatric failure to thrive syndrome, and depression, 57
Grief, morbid grief, 56

H
Haloperidol, for difficult behavior, 82
Hiccup, treatment of, 110
History of patient, components of, 16–17
Home care, 94–99, 185–187
caregiver support, 98–99
care process, 95–98
conference about care, 97
contraindications to, 97–98
and crisis situation, 96
doctors, 95
notes on, 185–187

positive aspects of, 94, 96
types of, 94
Huntington's disease, and
    dementia, 50
Hydrochlorothiazide, 25
Hydromorphone, for pain control,
    108
Hypertension, 27

I

Imipramine, for incontinence, 43
Incompetence
    capability of patient, 115–116
    and living will, 116
    substitute decision making, 116
Incontinence, 17, 39–53, 162–165
    behavioral incontinence, 41
    continuous dribbling
        incontinence, 41
    evaluation of, 41–43, 162
    nondrug treatments, 25, 43–44
    notes on, 162–165
    stress incontinence, 40
    surgical procedures, 43
    treatment of, 43–44
    urge incontinence, 40–41
Infection
    and dementia, 50
    of pressure sores, 74
Instrumental activities of daily
    living (IADL), 13

L

Lifestyle, and aging, 7–8
Living will, 116
Local anesthetics, for pain
    control, 109
Lorazepam, 82
Loxapine, 25, 80
    for difficult behavior, 82

M

Marijuana, for nausea, 110
Medical director, of nursing
    home, 103
Medication side-effects
    constipation, 71
    delirium, 49

for depression, 56
difficult behavior, 79–80
Mercy killing, 114
Metabolic imbalance, and
    delirium, 48–49
Metoclopramide, for nausea, 109
Mobility, 33–37, 159–161
    evaluation of, 17, 34–35
    failure, causes of, 35–36, 154
    normal mobility, 33–34
    notes on, 159–161
    treatment of mobility failure,
        36–37
Moclobemide, for depression, 58
Morbid grief, 56
Morphine
    for pain control, 108
    for shortness of breath, 110
Musculoskeletal system,
    evaluation of, 18

N

Narcotics, for pain control, 109
Nausea, treatment of, 109–110
Neuroleptics
    for difficult behavior, 82
    for pain control, 109
    for shortness of breath, 110
Nifedipine, for incontinence, 43
Nitrous oxide, for pain control,
    109
Nonsteroidal anti-inflammatory
    drugs (NSAIDs), 25
    for pain control, 109
Nortriptyline, for depression, 58–
    59
Nursing home care, 100–105,
    188–190
    characteristics of, 101–102
    and cognitive impairment, 100–
        101, 102
    and decision making, 101–102
    doctor in, 102–103, 105
    documentation, 104–105
    health interventions, 102, 103–
        104
    medical director, role of, 103
    notes on, 188–190

and relocation stress, 101
special care units, 101
types of facilities, 100
Nutritionist, 90

O
Opioids, for pain control, 108–109
Orthostatic hypotension, 18, 26, 36
Oxazepam, for difficult behavior, 82
Oxybutinin, for incontinence, 43
Oxycodone, for pain control, 108

P
Pain, 107–109
  and depression, 56
  and difficult behavior, 79
  drugs for, 108–109
  pain scales, 108
  total pain, meaning of, 108
Palliative care, 107–110, 191–193
  for constipation, 110
  for cough, 110
  for diarrhea, 110
  for hiccup, 110
  for nausea/vomiting, 109–110
  notes on, 191–193
  for pain control, 107–109
  for shortness of breath, 110
Parkinson's disease, 25, 28, 35, 36, 65
  and dementia, 50
  and depression, 56
Paroxetine, for depression, 58
Pharmacist, 90
Phenothiazines, for nausea, 109
Phenytoin
  for difficult behavior, 83
  for hiccup, 110
Physical examination, components of, 17–19
Physicians
  home care, 95
  nursing home, 102–103, 105
Physiotherapist, 90

Polypharmacy, 26, 156–157
  nature of, 24
Prescribing, and elderly, 23–30, 156–158
  challenges in, 23–24
  and compliance, 27, 28
  cost factors, 28
  guidelines for, 24–28
  notes on, 156–158
  and polypharmacy, 24, 26
  reducing medication, meaning of, 26–27
Pressure sores, 73–75, 178–179
  causes of, 73–74
  prevention of, 74–75
Propantheline, for incontinence, 43
Proprioception, 34
Pseudoephedrine, for incontinence, 43
Psychiatric history, 17
Psychosocial aging, 7, 150
Pyrexia, 49

R
Radiation, for pain control, 109
Relocation stress, and nursing home care, 101
Risperidone, problems with, 82

S
Salbutamol nebulizer, for cough, 110
Scopolamine, for nausea, 110
Selective serotonin reuptake inhibitors for depression, 58
  and difficult behavior, 79–80
Senior citizen's housing, 100
Sertraline, for depression, 58
Shortness of breath, treatment of, 110
Short Portable Mental Status Questionnaire, 15, 47, 51
Skilled nursing facilities, 100
Social isolation, 5
Social supports, 15–16
Social workers, 90–91
Stress incontinence, 40–43

Substance abuse, evaluation of,
    17, 18, 154
Suicide, and age, 54

T
Tacrine, and Alzheimer's disease,
    50
Team management, 89–93, 183–
    184
  care process, 91–92
  in comprehensive geriatric
    assessment (CGA), 11–12,
    91–92
  informal team members, 90
  notes on, 183–184
  team, meaning of, 89
  team conflict, 92
  team members, 90
  team roles, 90–91
  troubleshooting by, 92–93
Temazepam
  for difficult behavior, 82
  side effects, 82
Terazosin, for incontinence, 43
Thioridazine, side effects, 82
Transcutaneous electric nerve

  stimulation (TENS), 25
Trauma, and dementia, 49
Tricyclic antidepressants, for
    depression, 58–59

U
Urge incontinence, nature of, 40–
    41
Urinary incontinence. *See*
    Incontinence

V
Valproate, for difficult behavior,
    83
Vascular dementia, 49
Venlafaxine, for depression, 59
Vitamin deficiencies, and
    dementia, 50

W
Wernicke's encephalopathy, 49
Withdrawal, from alcohol, 17, 63
Women
  as caregivers, 98–99
  outliving men, 5